Off the Wall
Exercises for Climbers

Lisa M. Wolfe

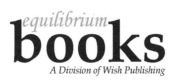

equilibrium
books
A Division of Wish Publishing

LCCN: 2005927149

Edited by Heather Lowhorn
Editorial assistance provided by Dorothy Chambers
Cover designed by Phil Velikan
Cover photography and interior photography provided by Lisa M. Wolfe

Printed in the United States of America
10 9 8 7 6 5 4 3 2 1

Published in the United States by
Equilibrium Books, A Division of Wish Publishing
P.O. Box 10337
Terre Haute, Indiana 47801, USA
www.wishpublishing.com

Distributed in the United States by
Cardinal Publishers Group

For my Dad,
who has helped me to climb to great heights!

TABLE OF CONTENTS

Chapter 1
Overview of Strength, Flexibility and Cardiovascular Training

Do you ever find yourself stuck on the climbing wall, hanging by the end of your rope? Willing your fingers to hold on and your heart to stop pounding? Do you silently wish for strength? Well, your wish can come true. But first you'll have to climb down and spend some time training off the wall.

Don't panic at the suggestion to get off the wall. There's a saying in climbing circles: "The best training for climbing is climbing." We need to move beyond that and realize that the time you spend training your body off the wall can lead to improvements on the wall. As a climber, you already know that climbing uses all of the muscles of the body. After climbing a difficult wall, you've probably discovered muscles you didn't even know that you had. Specific training can improve the weakest links that are holding back your climbing performance. You may have strong arms, for example, but lack the grip strength to hold you to the wall. Training off the wall will give you advancements in your climbs and could mean the difference between climbing a 5.7 and a 5.11 or help move you from solely top-roping into some lead climbing. Still not convinced? Give off-the-wall training a try anyway. It isn't going to hurt you, and you might just be surprised by the results. What have you got to lose?

By working to strengthen and stretch the muscles of the body, condition the heart and lungs, and improve mind focus and concentration, climbing can be all that you want it to be and more. The feeling of accomplishment you get when reaching the top of a climb can be yours every time. The body control that it takes to overcome challenges while climbing leads to improved self-esteem. You can enhance this body control and improve power through a workout regimen that includes strength, flexibility and cardiovascular exercise. So climb down for a little while and learn how off-the-wall training can help you stay on the wall longer and be stronger.

Strength Training

Climbing relies on all the muscles of the body, so it makes sense that a strength-training program can improve the ability to climb and lead to a more enjoyable experience with less muscular fatigue. Muscles respond to resistance by increasing muscle fiber size and strength. The strength of ligaments and tendons surrounding the muscles is also increased. Muscular adaptation occurs quickly. Even if muscles have never been exposed to strength training, the results will be seen within four to six weeks. On the flip side, muscle degeneration occurs even more quickly without appropriate stimulis, within approximately two weeks. The stimulus given to the muscles must be continuously changed. After six to eight weeks of the same workout, the body will stop responding in the same way. New challenges must be given in order to see improvements in strength.

In order to keep challenging your muscles, sample workouts are included at the end of each chapter. I suggest spending a week with each workout and then rotating the weeks in order of your preference. That way, the body will be challenged continuously. You will find some exercises that you enjoy more than others, and it is acceptable to participate in your favorite exercises every week if you choose. However, reserve the easier weeks of training for the periods of more intense climbing.

You do not need to purchase expensive exercise equipment or gym memberships in order to get an effective workout. Muscles respond to any type of resistance whether it's a dumbbell, resistance exercise band, full milk jugs, rocks or the body itself. Muscles cannot see whether you are using the hottest new equipment; they respond to the increased tension. Focus on performing the exercise, not on having perfect equipment.

The body needs 24 hours of rest between sessions to recover from a workout, but you can strengthen different muscle groups on different days. In general, the exercises should be performed two to three times per week to build up muscular strength and endurance. Strength training will be discussed in detail in Chapters 2 and 3.

Plyometric exercises are strength-training exercises that have their roots in jump training. Plyos link strength with speed of movement to produce power. The exercises begin with the muscles in a slightly elongated or stretched position. The muscles quickly move into a shortening contraction. When muscles are repeatedly trained this way, the result is a more forceful movement for propelling the body. The muscles, tendons and nerve receptors increase their sensitivity to the movements and respond with increased power. This power is used in dynamic climbing moves which propel the body up toward the next hold. Plyometric-training exercises can be found in Chapter 8.

Flexibility

Climbing does not use muscle groups evenly. Every route is different and will excite the body in different ways. Some routes require a greater reach where flexibility is the key. Flexibility is the joint's ability to move through a full range of motion. This range of motion can be limited by genetics, structure, activity level or injury. A regular stretching routine counteracts these limiting factors and helps to balance muscle groups.

Stretching, very basically, involves overcoming resistance in a joint by applying force. Elongating the muscle fibers and connective tissue is the goal. To receive the most benefits from stretching, daily participation is best. A low-intensity, long-duration (15-30 second) stretch is favored to alleviate joint stiffness and muscular pain. The stretches are held in control with no bouncing in the stretch.

The body should be warm before stretching. Muscles are likened to a piece of plastic. If plastic is forced to bend while it is cold, it will snap. If plastic is warmed up first, it will gently bend. Muscles are the same. Stretching a muscle when it's cold could result in a tear or pull. Stretching a muscle when it's warm will allow for a deeper stretch, resulting in relief not pain. After the muscles are warm, stretching will facilitate muscular relaxation, tissue waste removal, the return of muscles to normal resting length and improved circulation.

Over-stretching can lead to instability at the joints. To decrease this vulnerability, I recommend a combination of stretching and strengthening exercises such as yoga. Yoga exercises are stretching and strengthening exercises performed in a sequence. Each pose counteracts the previous one to balance the body and provide intense stretching. The strength gains from yoga are felt throughout the body into the muscle stabilizers. This means we do not simply train the large muscle groups, but the smaller muscles as well.

Yoga also helps to focus the mind. The concentration in yoga is on breathing. This concentration focuses the mind on the task at hand. This concentration during yoga transfers to being on the wall. The mind will remember the intense focus experienced in yoga and will concentrate more easily when you are climbing.

More on flexibility and range of motion will be addressed in Chapter 6.

Cardiovascular

Climbing endurance can also be improved with a focus on cardiovascular, or aerobic, exercise. *Aerobic* means *with oxygen*. Aerobic exercises — such as walking, cycling, rollerblading, swimming — are long-term exercises to be performed for at least 30-45 minutes. They use the body's fat as the primary source of energy, allowing the body to sustain the exercise for the intended period of time. The heart rate remains elevated through the session. A simple way to determine if the heart rate is elevated in the correct zone is to perform the talk test. If you're unable to talk, you're working too hard. If you can sing, you're not working hard enough.

Training aerobically strengthens the heart, lungs and circulatory system. This strength aids in faster and longer climbs. Other benefits of cardiovascular exercise include lowered blood pressure, reduced stress, decreased body fat, increase in good cholesterol, decrease in bad cholesterol, weight loss, decreased symptoms of depression and reduced anxiety levels.

Cardiovascular exercise can be performed every day, but you'll need to do it at least three times a week in order to see improvements. It is important to pick exercises that are enjoyable. Varying the workout also helps to alleviate boredom and keep the body stimulated. More about cardiovascular exercise can be found in Chapter 7.

One form of cardiovascular and strength-training exercise is circuit training. Circuit training is based on time spent in different activities. The workout is set up in small stations, alternating a cardiovascular exercise with a strengthening exercise. Once or twice through all the stations completes the circuit. Time spent in each station can vary, but 1½ minutes in each works well. The workout can last anywhere from 20-60 minutes depending on the day's needs. This workout should also be performed with a day of rest in between to allow muscles recovery time. Sample circuit training workouts are in Chapter 9.

Chapter 2
Weight Training the Upper and Lower Body

Unlike Spider Man, we don't have the ability to stick to the wall. Yet, some climbers appear to do just that. What gives them this extra staying power? The answer is strong muscles and control over those muscles. Here are some simple off-the-wall exercises with terrific on-the-wall results.

A tip to keep in mind when strength training for climbing is to do as many bilateral exercises as possible. This means giving each arm or leg a weight of its own — for example, using a dumbbell in each hand instead of a barbell that goes between the hands. This way each muscle group gains the same strength improvements instead of being able to "cheat" and help the other side. The use of dumbbells also helps to strengthen the hands, fingers and wrists simply by grasping the weight.

Perform 2-3 sets of 8-10 repetitions of each of the following exercises.

Pull-ups

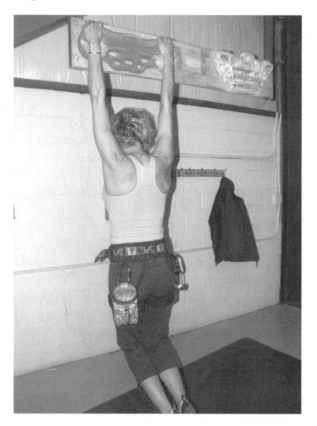

The most recommended exercise for the upper body has always been pull-ups, and for good reason. Pull-ups strengthen hands, arms, back, chest and the core. Another great benefit of pull-ups is there is no needed equipment. You just find something to hang from, whether a tree branch, door jamb, or bar, and the exercise can be modified for any level.

Place your hands on the bar with your palms facing away. The hands should be slightly wider than shoul-

Pull-ups

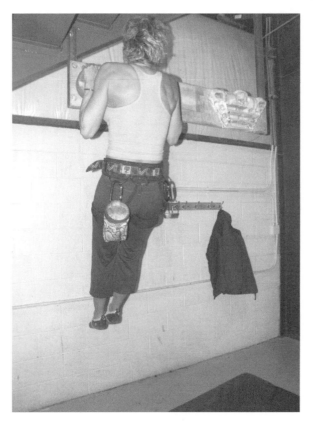

der-distance apart. Exhale, bend your elbows and pull your chin up over the bar. Inhale and slowly straighten the arms, releasing to the start position. For beginners: place feet on a chair. For intermediate: place one foot on a chair to a combination of half on and half off. For advanced: complete independent pull-ups, one arm pull-ups and endurance pull-ups.

Rows

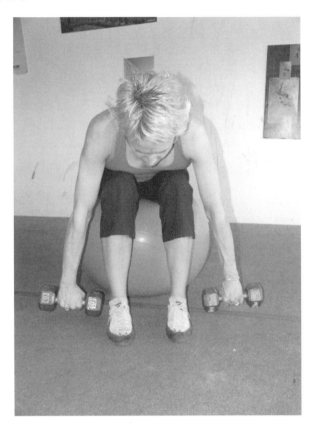

Rows are an excellent exercise to further strengthen the back. Sit in a chair or on a ball and hold a dumbbell in each hand. Bend forward from the hips, bringing your chest toward the tops of your legs. Allow your hands to drop next to your ankles and face your palms toward the back of the room. Exhale, and bending the

Rows

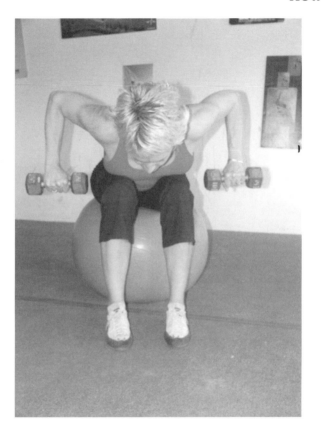

elbows, lift your hands up next to your hips. Squeeze your shoulder blades together. Inhale and straighten the arms, releasing the hands next to the ankles. This exercise targets the muscles between the shoulder blades to provide stability throughout the upper back. The stronger this area is, the less tension you'll hold there.

Strength Push

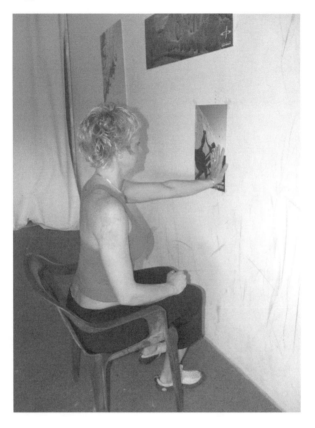

The strength push targets the lower back. Sit facing a wall, with your back straight and your chest lifted. Place your left hand onto the wall at shoulder level. Press forward, as if trying to push the wall away from you. Keep your core stable and do not twist into the movement. Hold this push for a count of 15, then repeat with your right arm. Continue alternating arms until you complete four cycles.

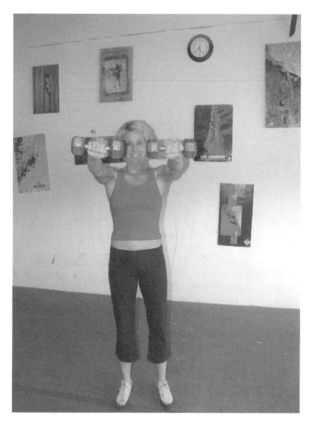

Front Raises, Side Raises and Rear Raises

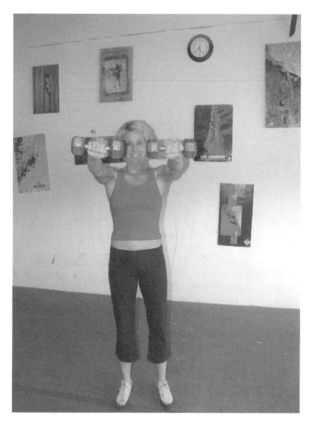

At the top of the upper body and used intensely for climbing are the shoulders. The shoulders are required for movements where the feet are not directly underneath you. The shoulder muscles have three distinct areas to them. It is important to train each independently for optimum results. The front, middle and rear deltoids (shoulders) act together to form a stable base from which the arms move. They also aid in posture. Most people regularly train the front and middle shoulder, but forget about the rear. To strengthen these three

Front Raises, Side Raises and Rear Raises

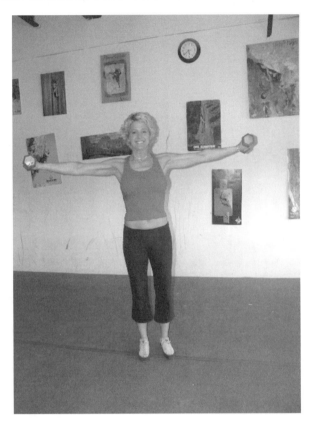

areas, we will be doing front raises, side raises and rear raises.

Stand tall with a dumbbell in each hand. Place your hands in front of the body with your palms facing toward the body. Bend the knees slightly to take pressure off the lower back. Exhale and with straight arms, raise the dumbbells up to the height of your eyes. Inhale and lower. Immediately following 8-10 repetitions, bring the arms to the sides of the body with the palms facing in. Exhale and with straight arms, raise the dumbbells out

Front Raises, Side Raises and Rear Raises

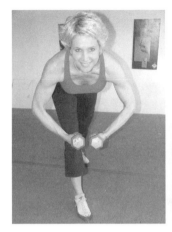

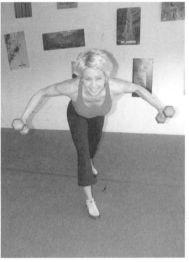

to the sides until the arms are parallel with the floor. Inhale and lower. Complete 8-10 repetitions here and then bring the right foot forward. Bend forward from the waist and place your arms in a position as if you're hugging a large barrel. Maintaining this arm position, exhale, separate your hands and press your elbows up toward the ceiling. Inhale and release to the start position. Complete a set of 8-10 repetitions. Repeat the entire sequence 2-3 times.

External Rotation

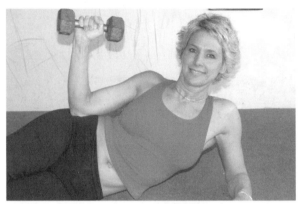

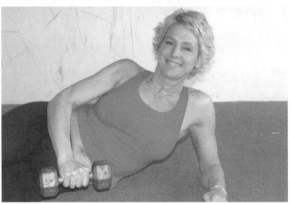

Deep within the shoulder lies a group of muscles re-
ferred to as the rotator cuff. Climbing puts strain on
these muscles which could result in a tear or a pull. To
ward off these injuries, use a rotation exercise to
strengthen the muscles. For external rotation, begin by
lying on your left side. Hold a dumbbell in your right
hand. The weight should be lighter than the one used
for the other shoulder exercises. Bend your right arm at
a 90-degree angle and allow your right elbow to rest on

your right hip with your hand raised toward the ceiling. Inhale and lower your hand to your belly button. Exhale and raise your hand back to the start position. Complete 2-3 sets of 8-10 repetitions. Repeat on the left arm.

Internal Rotation

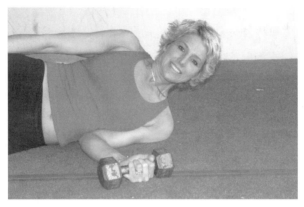

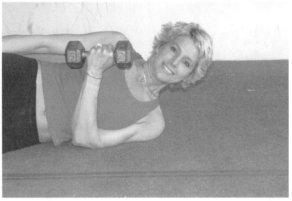

For internal rotation, remain lying in the same position as the external rotation, but this time bend the left arm at a 90-degree angle and rest the arm along the left side of the body. Hold the dumbbell in the left hand with the forearm flat on the base. Exhale and raise the left hand toward the right shoulder. Inhale and release the arm to the start position. Complete 2-3 sets of 8-10 repetitions. Repeat on the right arm.

Chest Fly

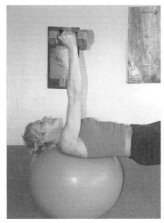

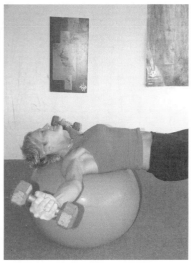

The chest also needs to be strengthened. The chest fly movement will increase strength down the center of the chest to aid in holding onto the wall with the arms extended out to the sides. Begin by lying on your back with a dumbbell in each hand. Straighten your arms toward the ceiling with the palms facing toward each other. Keep a slight bend in the elbows, inhale and open the arms out to the sides. Exhale and use the chest to return the arms to the starting position.

Push-ups

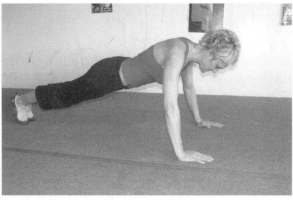

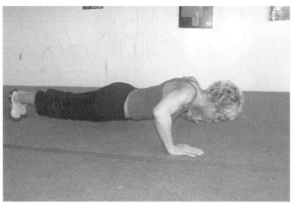

Push-ups are another complete upper-body exercise. Begin on your hands and knees. Place your hands on the floor, shoulder-distance apart. Straighten your legs behind you with your toes on the floor. Tighten the stomach and keep the spine straight. Inhale, bend your elbows and lower your chest toward the floor. Exhale, straighten your arms and return to the starting position.

Dumbbell Bicep Curl

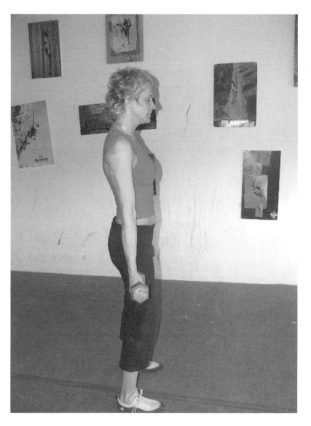

To strengthen the arms, we need to think about the body in its anatomical position. This is standing tall, with arms along the sides and the palms facing forward. The biceps muscle, the front of the upper arm, has two heads to it, hence the name "bi-ceps." For effective strengthening of this muscle, we need to train both heads. This is accomplished by changing the hand position.

Dumbbell Bicep Curl

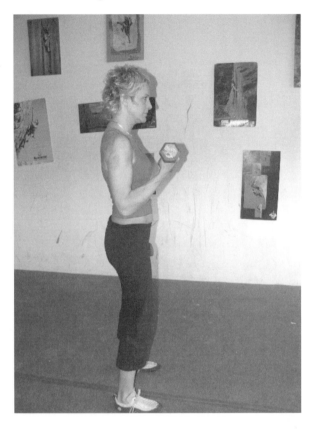

For the first position (with the palms facing up) stand or sit with your arms at your sides. Hold a dumbbell in each hand with your palms facing away from your body. Exhale and raise the palms toward the shoulders, keeping your elbows tight to your rib cage. Inhale and slowly lower the palms.

Reverse Curl

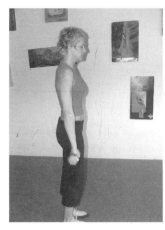

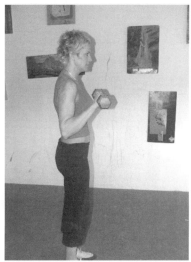

For the second position (with the palms facing down), stand tall with a dumbbell in each hand. Begin with your arms straight down and palms facing toward your body. Exhale and lift the hands toward the shoulders, keeping the palms facing the floor. Inhale and slowly lower the hands.

Dips

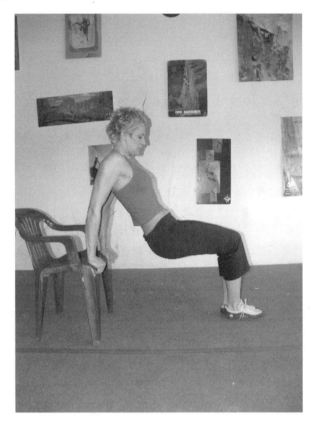

The triceps, the back of the upper arms, have three heads to the muscle, hence the name "tri-ceps." In order to strengthen this muscle, we need to train all three heads by changing the hand position. For the first hand position, sit on a ball, bench or chair. Place your palms next to your hips. Walk your feet away from the base,

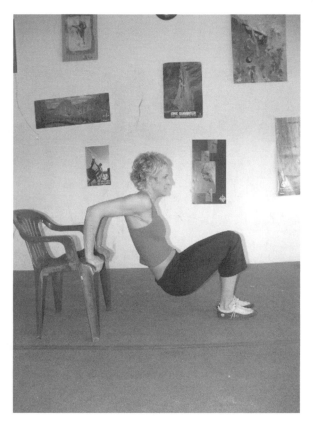

Dips

leaving your hips suspended in the air. Inhale and lower your hips toward the ground by bending your elbows behind the body to a 90-degree angle. Exhale and raise the hips by straightening the arms. To increase the intensity, straighten the legs or lift one leg toward the sky.

Kickbacks

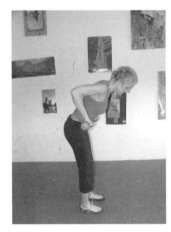

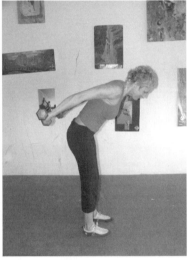

For the second hand position, stand tall with a dumb-bell in each hand. Bend forward slightly from your waist, lifting the elbows higher than the back. Turn your palms to face backward. (Palms can also face forward for increased intensity). Exhale and straighten your arms lifting the weights out behind the body. The palms should now be facing toward the floor. Inhale and bend the elbows, releasing back to the starting position.

Skull Crushers

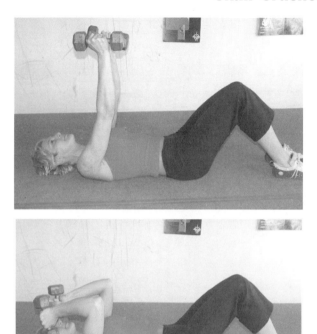

Another name for this exercise is the French curl. Begin by lying on your back with a dumbbell in each hand. Straighten your arms toward the ceiling and face your palms toward each other (the third hand position). Inhale and bend the elbows, bringing the weights toward the sides of your head. Exhale and straighten the arms back to the starting position.

Wide Leg Squats

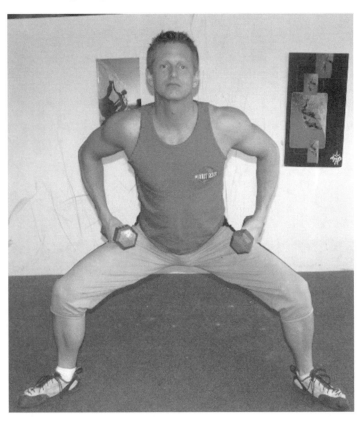

The legs provide the strength to move up the wall, especially in dynamic, jumping moves. Strong legs can make the difference between landing a hold and missing one. Using the legs for the movements saves the arms and hands from doing the majority of the effort. The stronger our legs, the more energy we save while on the wall. That will lead to faster and more frequent climbing. For wide leg squats, stand with legs wider than shoulder-distance apart. Bend your knees and turn the knees and toes slightly out to the sides. Inhale, bend your knees and lower your hips. Keep the weight of the body pressing through the heels. On an exhale, straighten your legs but keep a slight bend in the knee. You can use the weight of the body or add dumbbells held over the thighs. The quadriceps are especially strengthened with this exercise. Keeping the legs wide also aids in strengthening the inner thighs which help to keep the hips pressed into the wall while climbing.

Sumo Squat

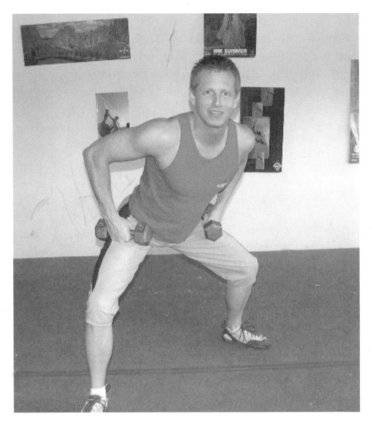

Begin standing in a wide-legged squat position. Place your hands on your upper thighs, resembling a sumo wrestler. These are squats with movement. Pick up your right foot and walk forward. Pick up your left foot and continue the walk. Continue alternating as you walk across the room, keeping your rear low, your knees bent and your back straight.

Stiff-legged Dead Lifts

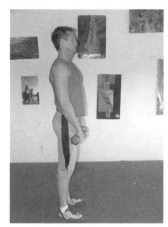

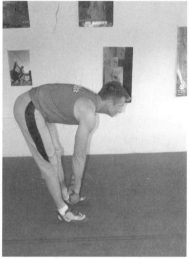

This strengthens the hamstrings. Stand tall with feet hip-distance apart. Hold a dumbbell in each hand with your palms facing toward your body. Inhale and bend forward from the waist. Keep your spine straight, stomach pulled in and look straight ahead. Only bend forward to a point where you can still look ahead. If the head begins to drop down, pull out of the exercise. On an exhale, squeeze your backside to pull the body back to standing tall.

Lunge and Lift

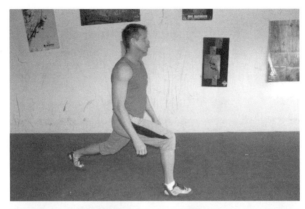

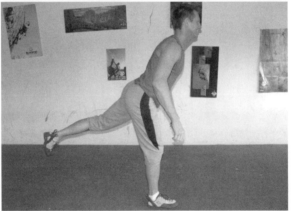

This exercise targets the gluteals. Begin in a lunge position with the right foot approximately two feet in front of the left. Inhale and bend the right knee to a 90-degree angle. Exhale and straighten the right leg while lifting the straight left leg off of the floor, squeezing with the behind. Lower the left leg and repeat. Repeat on the opposite leg.

Alternating Heel Lift/Toe Lift

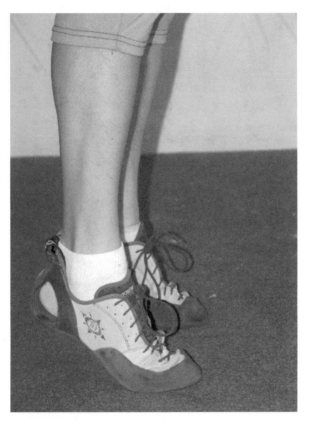

It's important to train the legs in various positions to mimic the poses on the wall. Your feet will not always be equal distance apart or directly underneath the body. They'll be staggered, crossed and possibly spread apart, depending on the climb. To help keep the toes on the wall and onto the small chips, the calves need to be strong. Having strong calf muscles also helps to protect the ankles. To strengthen the front and the back of the lower leg, an alternating heel lift/toe lift accomplishes

Alternating Heel Lift/Toe Lift

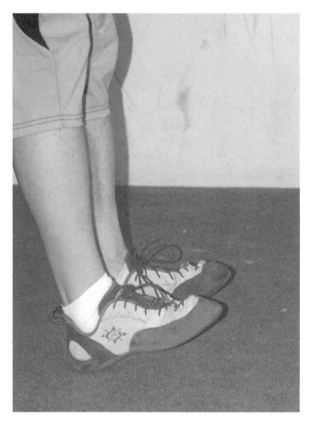

this. Stand tall holding a dumbbell in each hand. Exhale and lift your heels, coming up onto your toes. Inhale and roll back onto your heels, lifting your toes. Keep your spine straight and do not stick your rear out behind you: keep it underneath your body.

Seated Calf Raise

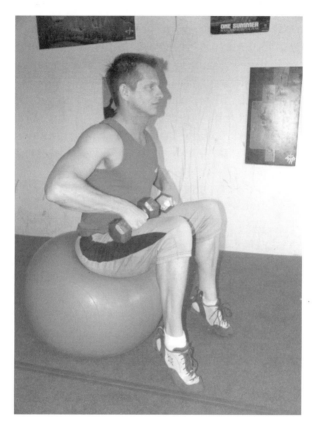

A seated calf raise strengthens the muscle deeper into the calf. Sit on a ball or in a chair. Keep your feet on the floor and bend your knees to a 90-degree angle. Hold dumbbells across your thighs and above the knees. Exhale and lift your heels, squeezing the backs of the legs. Inhale and lower the heels to the floor.

General Tips

One tip for successful training is to work from the larger muscle groups, such as the legs, chest and back, to the smaller muscle groups, including the arms, shoulders and calves. Training the larger groups first warms all of the muscles and leads to fewer injuries.

A strength-training routine should follow a day of climbing. To climb and strength train on the same day is a lot of work for the body. These workouts can be performed three days a week for maximum benefit, with a day of rest in between.

The amount of weight you use is based on how strong you are. Choose a weight that makes the last two repetitions of each set feel challenging. When you can do all three sets of 8-10 repetitions without a lot of effort, it's time to increase the amount of weight. A workout example using these exercises is shown in the following table:

Mon.	Tue.	Wed.	Thu.	Fri.
Pull-ups	REST or CLIMB	Seated Row	REST or CLIMB	Strength Push
Push-ups		Chest Fly		Push-Ups
Dumbbell Shoulder Raises		Rotator Cuff		Dumbbell Shoulder Raises
Dumbbell Bicep Curls		Reverse Dumbbell Curls		Dumbbell Bicep Curls
Dips		Kickbacks		Skull Crushers
Wide Leg Squats		Sumo Squats		Lunge and Lifts
Dead Lifts		Lunge and Lift		Dead Lifts
Rocking Calves		Seated Calf Raises		Rocking Calves

Chapter 3
Strength Training Hands and Wrists

Even if you've only climbed one time, you've noticed that the grip gives way before anything else. The most common injuries in climbing are to the hands and wrists. The fingers, in particular, take the brunt of the damage from climbing. It makes sense then, that improving the strength in your grip will improve your climbing. Strengthening exercises can prepare the hands for the excessive demands of climbing and aid in injury prevention.

The hands are used in various positions on the wall. It's not always a grab to pull you up. At times it will be a push against the opposite wall or a push underneath to boost yourself up to the next hold. The hands are used on under-clings with the palms facing up, or angled for sloping movements. The hands can also be held toward the side of the body for any leaning movements. You can train the hands to be stronger in all of these positions.

Hanging

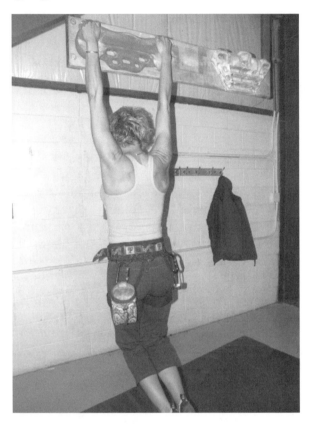

A typical route takes less than four minutes to complete, yet if the forearms give out before this, you'll be left hanging. Speaking of hanging, that is the best way to improve forearm strength for climbing. Find a bar, a branch, or a piece of wood to hang from. Hang until your hands, forearms and grip completely fail. You can vary the bend in the elbow to train the muscles in different positions. Begin with a straight arm hang, and progress to hanging with the elbows bent at a 90-degree angle. From there, work to holding the arms at an angle between straight and 90 degrees. It's important to build up that endurance so the muscles will remember that sensation. Muscles have memory, and they will remember hanging in this position.

Dumbbell Lift

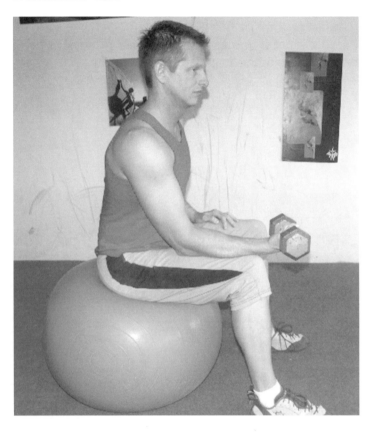

The very act of strength training, holding onto a dumbbell or barbell, challenges the muscles of the forearms, wrists and hands. For specific forearm and wrist strength, use a dumbbell lift. Sit and rest your forearm on your upper leg. Hold a dumbbell in your hand with the palm facing up and allow only the hand to extend beyond the knee. Exhale and raise the palm toward the sky. Inhale and lower the hand, slowly rolling the dumbbell out toward the fingertips.

Dumbbell Lift

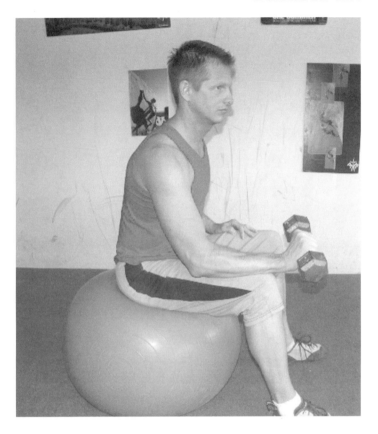

Then flip the palm over, grasp the dumbbell in your hand and as you exhale raise the back of the hand toward the sky. Inhale and lower the hand. Aim for complete range of motion. Raise and lower the hand as high and low as possible. This will activate the most muscle fibers.

Dead Hanging

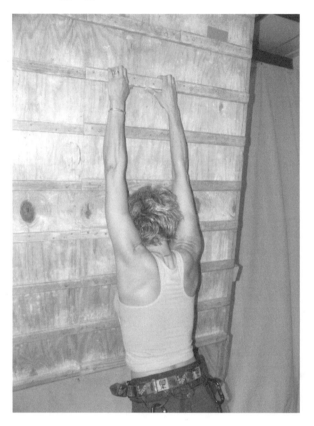

Dead hanging from the fingertips can also be used. You'll need a finger board or campus board with various widths of finger holds. Begin by hanging for 2-4 seconds and build up to hanging for 10-12 seconds. Continue to challenge your fingers by choosing holds that are increasingly smaller. It is helpful to train one arm at a time. This hanging exercise can be done with one hand until fatigued, and then followed with the other. Try for three sets of these hangs in order to see improvements.

Hand Exerciser

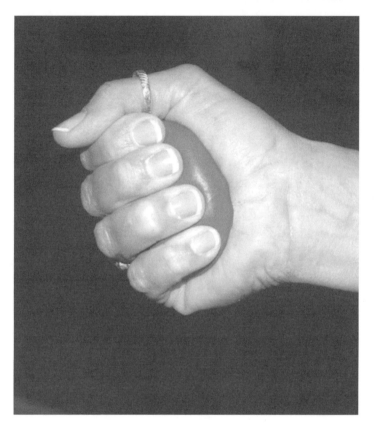

Spring-loaded hand exercisers or stress balls that you squeeze will aid in training for hand and grip strength. The nice thing about these is their ease of use. While riding in a car, you can train one hand at a time. The goal is to work up to squeezing for 20 minutes. This will increase strength and endurance in the forearms. With a ball, you can place it between each finger and squeeze the fingers together for added strength.

Rubber Band

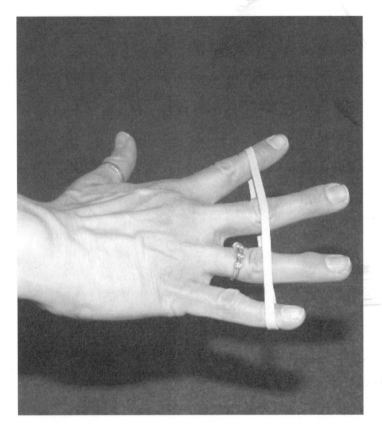

Another simple exercise for finger strength is to use a rubber band. Place the fingers inside of the rubber band and spread them apart against the resistance of the band. Slowly release the fingers together, keeping them in line with one another.

Wrist Flexion

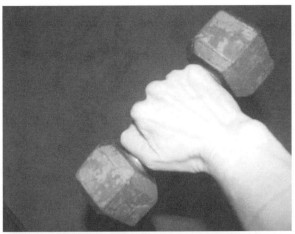

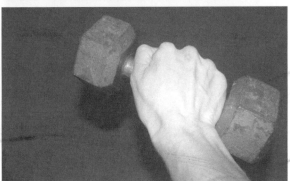

A side movement to the hands, flexion, will also help to strengthen the wrists. Holding a dumbbell in the hands with the palms facing toward the floor, move the thumb side of the hands toward the forearms. Then, reverse the direction and move the little finger side of the hands toward the forearms. Repeat for 8-10 repetitions in each direction. Maintain a straight line through the forearms and wrists to provide stability for the exercise.

Rotating the Wrist

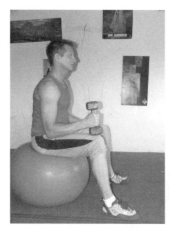

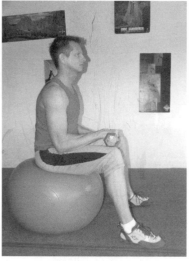

Turn the hand so that the palm is facing toward the midline of the body. One head of the dumbbell rests on the leg, and the other head is on top of the hand. Using a windshield wiper movement, lower the top head of the dumbbell toward the leg with the palm facing down. Then reverse the movement to lay the head of the dumbbell toward the leg with the palm facing up. The elbow stays stationary and the movement is slow and controlled.

Wrist Circles

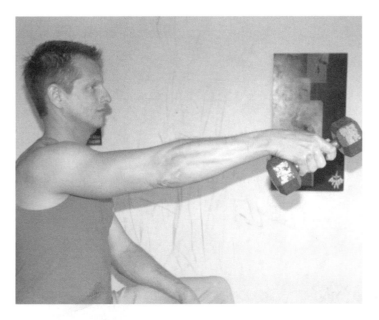

Begin by holding onto the dumbbell as if it were a magic wand. Extend your arm out straight with your hand level to the shoulder. Face one head of the dumbbell away from the body and one toward the body with the palm facing inward. Rotate the dumbbell in a clockwise motion, completing 10 circles. Next, rotate the dumbbell in a counterclockwise motion for 10 circles.

Push-up Variations

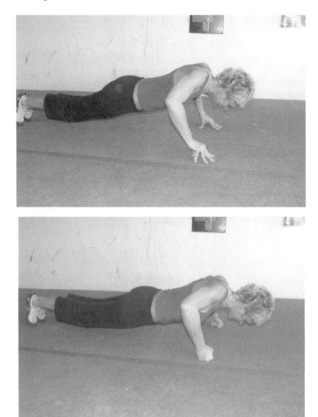

Strengthening the wrists can be incorporated through-out the other strength-training exercises. For example, instead of resting on the palms of the hands when do-ing push-ups, rest on the fingertips to strengthen the wrists and fingers. Push-ups can also be done on a fisted hand with the knuckles on the floor. This keeps the wrists strong and active.

Add one or two of these forearm and wrist exercises to the workout program for overall benefits. Simply strengthening the forearms alone will improve your climbing abilities. Adding forearms to a complete body workout will dramatically improve your climbing abilities.

In order to prevent injuries, we must remember the limitations of the fingers. When we incorporate the entire body into climbing, we reduce the amount of work needed from the fingers. The most common reason for finger injuries is overuse. By strengthening the muscles we can help to avoid this problem, too.

An example of how to add these exercises into your weekly routine is shown in the following table:

Mon.	Tue.	Wed.	Thu.	Fri.
Dumbbell Forearm Lifts Rubber Band Exercises	REST Or CLIMB After climbing, hanging exercise	Wrist Rotation Wrist Circles	REST or CLIMB After climbing, spring-loaded finger exercise	Hanging Fingertip Push-up

Chapter 4
Core and Balance Training

Four out of five adults experience back pain in their lifetimes. Impairment is most prevalent in the 45- to 64-year-old age group. The problem becomes chronic for 5 to 10 percent of sufferers. Acute back pain recovery can take from three days to six weeks. Unfortunately, once a back injury occurs, a person is four times more likely to re-injure it.

Why is the back so susceptible to injury? For the answer, let's look at how the back is constructed. The spinal column consists of 33 vertebrae stacked upon each other, 26 of which are movable. Abdominal and back muscles support the spine. If these muscles are weak or inflexible, the spine is pulled in an unnatural direction, usually resulting in pain. Some causes of back pain are:

- inactivity
- lack of flexibility in the hamstrings, causing a tight lower back
- weak abdominal muscles
- overweight body
- poor posture
- lifting improperly (i.e., without bending the legs)
- sleeping face down
- physical injury
- age, wear and tear.

Core, abdominal and back exercises improve the strength of the stomach and back and improve the flexibility of the spine. A healthy spine helps you to be more aware of your body in all of its various positions.

The core is used when lifting your feet up onto the wall at the beginning of any climb. When bouldering, especially when the hands and feet are on a wall over the top of the body, the core is working to hold the feet to the wall. A strong core will aid in keeping the body on the wall, especially when climbing overhangs. When your core is strong, less energy is used from the other muscles to keep you on the wall. This core provides a stable base from which all of your movements originate.

Any sideways leans off a hold require core strength to keep the torso stable. Sideways leans allow for a diagonal reach toward a hold. Reaching for footholds also requires torso stability to keep the hands in place. Strengthening the core brings greater awareness to that area. This will bring greater control when ascending a climb.

In order to keep a healthy and functional core:
• increase flexibility of the lower back, hip flexors and hamstrings
• build strength in abs, obliques and erector spinae
• maintain a neutral spinal posture throughout the day
• Use active sitting (i.e., sitting on a stability ball) instead of passive chair sitting.

Transverse Abdominis

Begin by training the transverse abdominis — the deepest layer of muscle tissue in the abdomen. The transverse abdominis maintains core stability, helping provide support to the spine, rib cage and pelvis. Train the transverse abdominis by tightening the stomach. This tightening can be accomplished by mimicking the feeling of squeezing into a tight pair of pants. Keep this muscle pulled tight throughout the exercises.

Rectus Abdominis and Obliques

The rectus abdominis is the muscle that travels up the center of the abdomen. This muscle allows us to bend forward and helps to support the abdominal cavity. Other muscles that aid in supporting the abdominal cavity and the external and internal oblique muscles. These allow the body to twist and bend sideways.

Traditional, full sit-ups utilize the muscles of the abdomen, but also involve the tops of the legs and compromise the back. Crunches are better, and crunches on the ball are better still. The rectus abdominis, external and internal obliques can be trained with the following exercises:

Trunk Curl

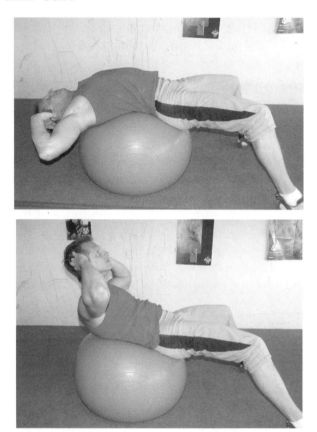

Sit on the ball and walk your feet forward until the ball is beneath the small of your back. Place your hands behind your head or crossed on top of your chest (this is the easier option). Press your lower back into the ball, curling the rib cage toward the pelvis. Return to the starting position.

Standing Pelvic Tilt

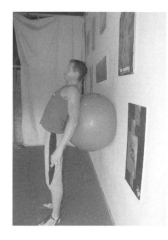

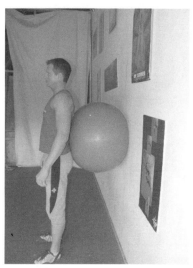

Begin by standing with the ball between a wall and the small of your back. Bend your knees and space your legs hip-distance apart. Arch the back around the ball. Using the abdominal muscles, flatten the back by pulling the hips toward the rib cage, then slowly release to the starting position.

Side Planks

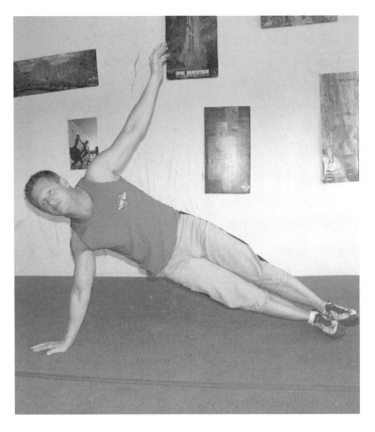

Begin by lying on your right side with your legs straight and stacked upon each other. Place your right hand onto the floor directly underneath your shoulder. Raise your left arm toward the ceiling. Exhale and lift your hips off the floor, shifting your weight onto the side of your right foot. Hold for a count of 15-20, then switch to the opposite side. For more advanced movement, hold each side for one breath, with a quick switch in between. This exercise strengthens the sides, abdominals, back, arms and shoulders.

Reverse Trunk Twist

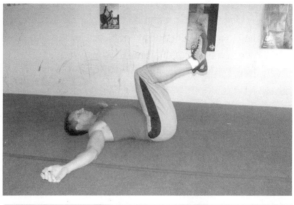

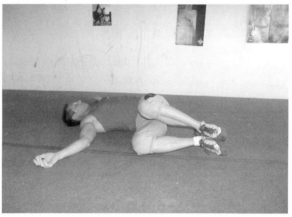

Begin by lying on your back with your arms out to the sides at shoulder level and your legs 90 degrees from the floor. Inhale and lower your legs to the right, touching the floor with the outside foot. Exhale and raise your legs back to the start position. Inhale and lower your legs to the left and touch the floor with the outside foot. Exhale and return to start. For an advanced movement, straighten the knees. Concentrate on keeping your shoulders pressed down into the floor. This exercise strengthens the sides and front of the abdominal muscles.

Erector Spinae

The erector spinae is the largest back muscle. It extends on each side of the spinal column, from the pelvic region to the cranium. Erector spinae strength and endurance are necessary for a healthy back and good posture. Use the following exercises to train the erector spinae:

Spinal Balance

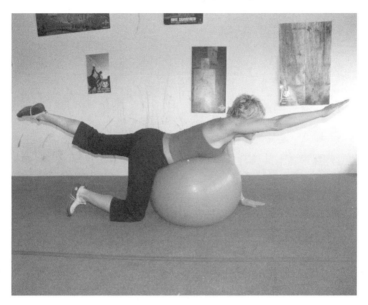

Lie face down with the ball in the center of your abdomen, and with hands and knees shoulder-width apart on the ground. To maintain this position, you may need to adjust the ball size accordingly. Keep the spine in a neutral position by holding the abdominal muscles tight. Slowly raise one arm, while raising the opposite leg to hip level. Return to the starting position and repeat, using the other arm and leg. Concentrate on reaching away from the body, through the fingers and the toes, and lengthening the spine.

Leg Lifts

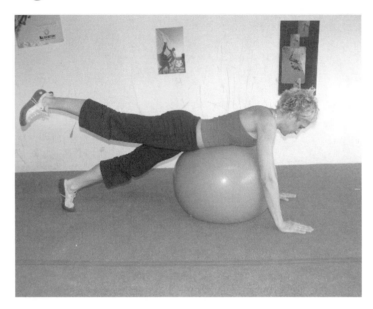

Working in the same position with your stomach on the ball, keep hands on the floor and straighten your legs slightly so your toes touch the ground. Lift one leg to hip level, keeping the spine straight and abdomen contracted. Lower the leg to the floor and repeat with the opposite leg. For a more challenging exercise, lift both legs at the same time.

Arm Lifts

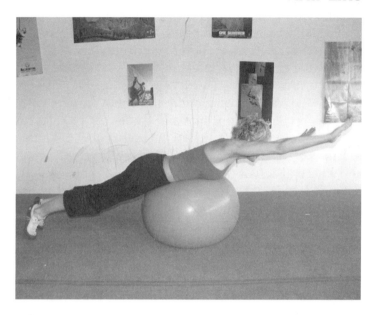

Working in the same position with your stomach on the ball, slightly bend the knees and keep your toes on the floor. Extend your arms straight out in front of you, so that you make a straight line from your hands to the base of your spine. From this starting position, lift your chest off the ball while keeping your arms in the same position, extending your spine. Return to the starting position.

Balance

Quite simply, balance is the ability to maintain body position over a base of support. Even simple everyday movements such as walking require balance. When walking or running we are consistently alternating between losing and regaining our balance. Our ankles provide the corrective action for these movements. Each time the body shifts position and comes out of balance, muscles are activated to bring the body back into equilibrium. If we increase the balance challenge, the hips and knees also help adjust for balance. Problems with balance are often the result of a weak core. Training the balance system and the core of the body provide a stable base for the arms and legs.

Balance on the wall is especially important when shifting weight from one foot to the other. When balance is strong, the hands don't have to work as hard to hold you to the wall, and you don't waste energy with excess motion. Your movements appear graceful.

Since your center of gravity shifts often when you are on the wall, it's important to train for balance in a variety of positions. The good news is that balance responds quickly to a training program. To begin, do the exercises as stated. When you've accomplished that, close your eyes while doing the exercises for a further challenge. You can also change the surface, such as moving to grass instead of a hard floor, or standing on exercise mats, to increase the challenge of the exercises. Another good tip is to vary the time of day the exercises are performed.

The use of the stability ball will help to train your body to function as a unit. The entire body works together to keep you on that ball, which activates more muscle fibers. The following are great balance exercises that utilize the stability ball.

Kneeling on the Ball

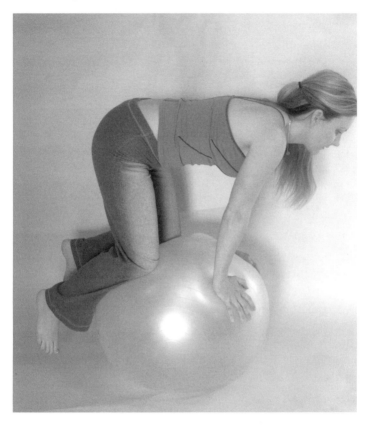

Place the ball on the floor. Facing the ball, place both hands on the opposite side of it. Rest your knees on the ball and slowly roll up until you can lift one or both feet off the ground. For a more advanced exercise, lift both hands up and balance solely with the knees on the ball. Maintain a strong stomach and a straight spine. Hold this position for a count of 30 and repeat 2-3 times.

Inner Thigh Balance

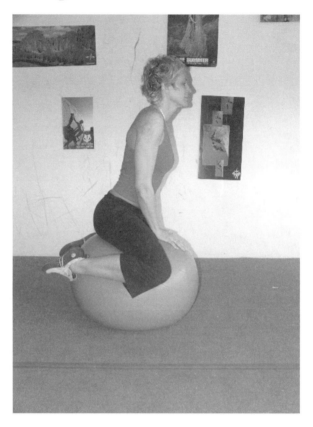

Place the ball on the floor. Approach the ball as if straddling a horse. Straddle the ball with knees pointing toward the floor and your feet behind your body with your toes into the floor. You may rest your hands on the ball between your knees as you lift your feet off the floor and balance. Squeeze your thighs toward each other and hold your stomach pulled in. Hold this position for a count of 30 and repeat 2-3 times.

Seated Balance (Feet Off the Floor)

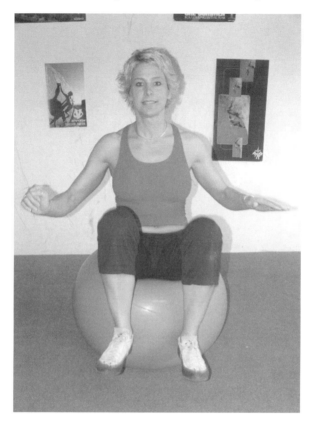

Sit on top of the ball. Lift your right leg with your knee bent and place your right foot on the ball. Tighten your stomach, lift your left leg and place your left foot on the ball. Maintain this balance for a count of 30, then repeat 2-3 times.

Stand on One Leg

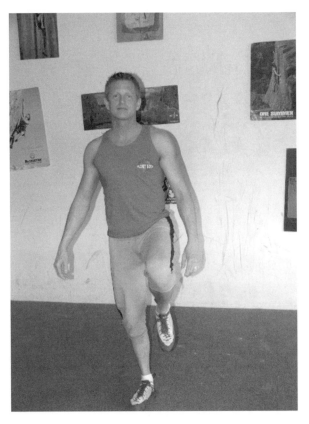

The use of the body alone can also provide opportunities to increase balance.

Simply standing on one leg can provide a balance challenge. Keeping the body tall, shift your weight onto your right leg. Slowly lift the left foot off the floor. Keep your arms at your sides and try not to sway. Hold for a count of 20, and then repeat on the left leg. To further increase the intensity, close your eyes.

One-Legged Reach

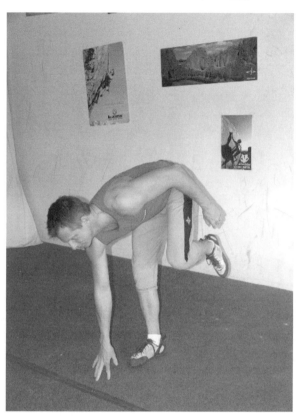

A one-legged reach takes standing on one leg to the next level. Stand tall and shift your weight onto your right leg. Inhale and lift the left foot behind the body as you reach down with your right hand to touch the floor in front of your right foot. Remember to hold the stomach in tight and keep the spine straight. Exhale and return to start, not setting the left foot down until you have completed 8-10 repetitions. Repeat on the left leg. Again, the intensity can be increased by closing your eyes.

One-Legged Squat

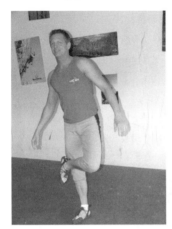

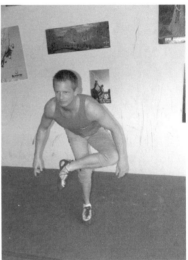

Stand tall and shift your weight onto your right leg. Lift the left foot and place it above the right knee. Look straight ahead, inhale and bend your right leg until it's at a 90-degree angle. Exhale, straighten your right leg and return to start. Perform 2-3 sets of 8-10 repetitions on both legs.

(Note: A balance board is a useful tool that can be purchased or made from wood. A balance tool will improve your control of balance, posture, stability and will awaken your equilibrium.)

Squats

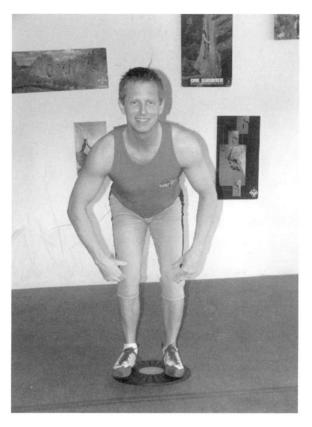

Place your feet on the balance board. Do not let the sides of the board touch the floor. Maintaining this balance look straight ahead, inhale and lower into a squat position. Do not bend the knees past a 90-degree angle. Exhale and straighten your legs back to the start position. Perform 2-3 sets of 8-10 repetitions on both legs.

Lunges

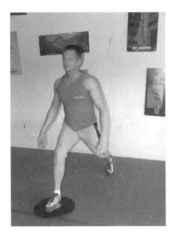

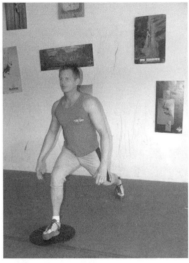

Stand with your right foot on the balance board and the left foot approximately two feet behind. Do not let the sides of the board touch the floor. Inhale and bend the knees lowering the hips. The right knee does not bend past a 90-degree angle. Exhale, straighten the legs and return to start. The challenge is to maintain a stable footing on the board without wobbling. Perform 2-3 sets of 8-10 repetitions on both legs.

Push-ups

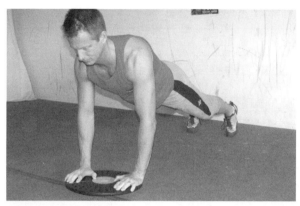

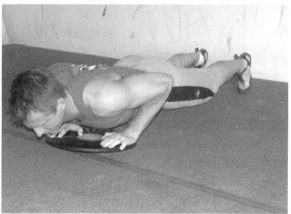

Place your hands on the balance board. Keep the sides from touching the ground. Straighten your legs behind you and let your toes rest into the floor. Tighten the stomach and keep the spine straight. Inhale, bend your elbows and lower your chest toward the board. Exhale, straighten your arms and release to the starting position. This exercise strengthens the upper body while building balance in the arms. Repeat for 8-10 repetitions and 2-3 sets.

The following table provides a sample core and balance training workout.

Mon	Tue	Wed	Thu	Fri
Trunk Curl Kneel on ball Side Planks One-Legged Standing Board Squats	REST or CLIMB	Pelvic Tilt Inner Thigh Balance Spinal Balance One-Legged Reach Board Lunges	REST or CLIMB	Rev. Trunk Twist Leg Lifts Seated Balance One-Legged Squat Push-ups

Chapter 5
Using Props

Stability Balls

A stability ball is a large, heavy-duty inflatable ball made to hold up to 700 pounds without bursting. Stability-ball training began in physical rehabilitation. Therapists used this unstable surface with their clients to rehabilitate existing injuries and to prevent new ones. Approximately 25 years ago, the stability ball was mainstreamed into the fitness world. Currently, we see stability balls used in homes as chairs and in schools for physical education classes.

The stability ball activates the core of the body in every movement. The unstable surface of the ball calls into play various muscles for stabilization. This allows for improved posture, less back pain and a flatter stomach.

The ball provides a round, moveable surface that is quite different for training than on a stable, flat bench. Since muscles are challenged to maintain their alignment and hold the body upright, one of the greatest benefits of ball training is the balance factor. Exercising on the ball also helps build postural endurance. All of these qualities – a strong core, balance and spinal endurance – are needed for a successful climb.

The balls come in different sizes and should be purchased according to height. For a person under 5 feet tall, a 45 cm ball will fit. For persons between 5 and 6 feet, a 55 cm ball will fit. The balls come with instructions and a foot pump to inflate. The firmer the ball is inflated, the more challenging the exercises will be. The softer the ball is, the easier the exercises will be. Use the ball on a smooth surface such as carpeting or a wood floor. The balls pick up dirt easily, so it is recommended that you keep them indoors. You should also wear shirts and pants to protect the skin. Repeat each exercise for 2-3 sets of 8-10 repetitions.

Two-Ball Pec Deck

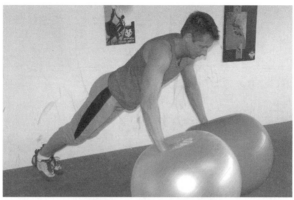

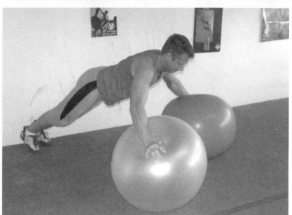

You'll need two balls for this exercise. Kneel in front of the balls and place one hand on each. Pull your stomach in tight and straighten your legs behind you, resting on the toes. Inhale and slowly separate your hands, rolling the balls out to the sides. Exhale and return the balls toward each other. Keep the movement slow and controlled and use the strength of the arms and chest to hold the balls stable.

Push-ups

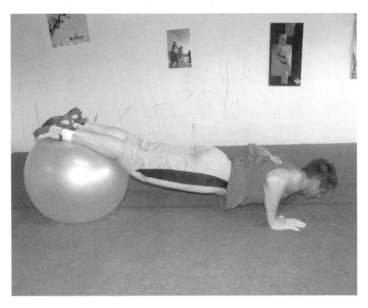

Lie face down and place the ball underneath the hips. Walk your hands out until the ball is between the knees and the ankles. The closer the ball is to the feet, the more challenging the exercise will be. Place hands on the floor, shoulder-distance apart. Inhale, bend the elbows and lower the chest toward the floor. Keep the spine straight and the stomach pulled in. Exhale, straighten your arms and return to start. The challenge here is keeping the body in a straight line while on an unstable surface.

One Legged Dead Lift

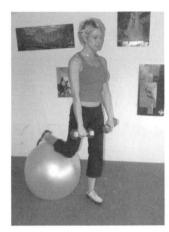

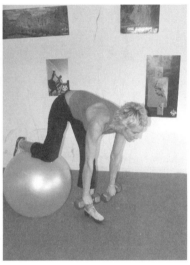

Stand with your back toward the ball. Bend your right knee and place the top of your right foot on the ball. Hold a dumbbell in each hand. Inhale and bend forward from the waist, keeping the dumbbells close to the body as the hands lower toward the floor. Look straight ahead to keep the spine in alignment. Exhale and, using the back side of the body, return yourself back to standing. This exercise strengthens the backs of the upper legs, hamstrings and the gluteals.

Wall Squat

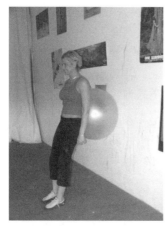

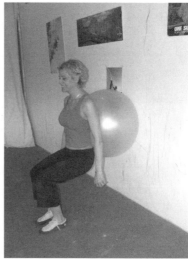

Stand with the ball between your back and a wall. Move your feet out away from the wall, so that you are leaning back into the ball. Inhale, bend your knees and lower your hips until the knees are bent at a 90-degree angle. Exhale, straighten your legs and return to start. Look straight ahead and keep the stomach pulled in while squatting. Keep your weight centered over your heels to protect your knees. This exercise strengthens the legs.

Tricep Lift

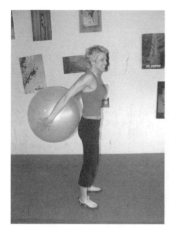

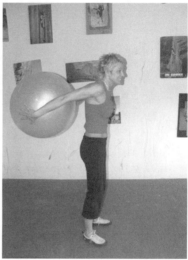

Stand and hold the ball behind your back with straight arms. Exhale and lift your hands toward the ceiling. Inhale and lower the ball. This exercise strengthens the arms and the back.

Oblique Lift

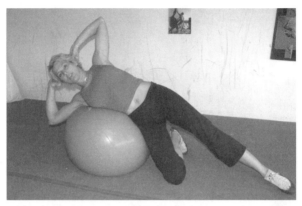

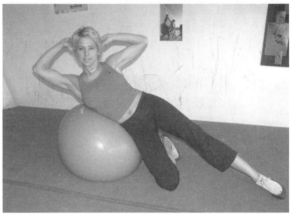

Kneel on the ground with the ball next to your right hip. Press your right hip into the ball, straighten your left leg and drape yourself over the top of the ball. Place your left hand behind your head and your right hand either on the ball or behind your head. Exhale and, using the muscles on the left side, raise your right side off the ball. Inhale and lower yourself over the ball. This strengthens the sides, also known as the obliques.

Foam Rollers

Foam rollers resemble the noodles that people use while floating in pools. The fitness rollers are thicker, and they don't have a hole in the middle. They are usually 6 inches in cylindrical diameter and can vary from 12-36 inches in length.

Training on rollers is like balancing on logs. There are tools used in rehabilitation to aid in balance, stability and muscle strength. For beginners, the rollers can be cut in half lengthwise so that the flat side can be faced down to provide a more stable base. The intermediate user can then turn the flat side up to provide a flat base for the feet before moving onto a full roller.

The very nature of rollers is an unstable surface. Training on this surface activates mental as well as physical coordination. Balance reactions are strengthened, and body awareness and muscular re-education are also improved. The mind is involved and becomes aware of every movement made in order to keep you on the roller. This mental strength also carries over onto the wall where the mind plays a large part in whether or not a climb is successful.

Squats

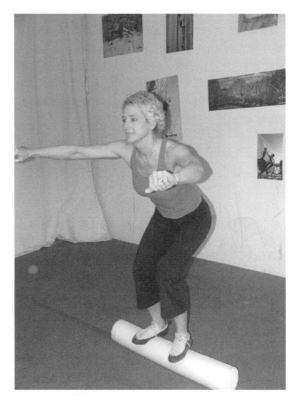

Place the roller horizontally on the floor in front of you. Step both feet onto the roller. Gain your balance, then inhale and bend the knees, lowering the hips into a squat. The knees should not exceed a 90-degree angle. Exhale and straighten your legs, returning to start. Look forward to help with balance. This exercise strengthens the lower body while improving balance.

Push-ups

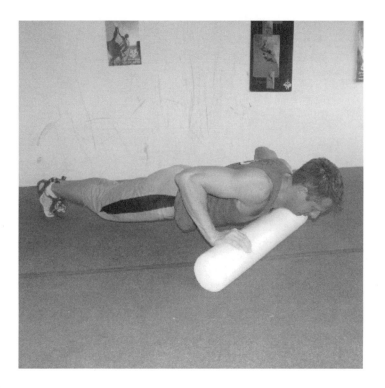

Place the roller horizontally on the floor in front of you. Kneel and place your hands on the roller. Your hands should be slightly wider than shoulder-distance apart. For a beginner, remaining on the knees is enough of a challenge. For an advanced exercise, straighten the legs and let your toes rest on the floor. Inhale and bend your elbows, lowering your chest toward the roller. Exhale, straighten your arms and return to the start position. These push-ups strengthen the chest, arms and back and improve hand strength and upper-body balance.

Bridge

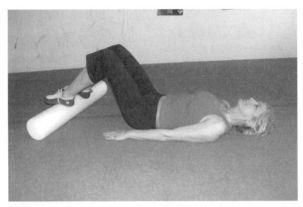

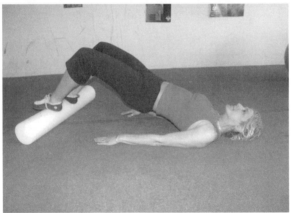

Place the roller horizontally on the floor. Lie on your back with your feet on the roller. The feet should be placed hip-distance apart with the knees and toes in alignment. With the roller approximately 2 feet from the body, inhale and raise your hips toward the ceiling, keeping your arms at your sides and your neck very still. You can hold for a count of 20 or lift and lower the hips for repetitions. For a more advanced exercise, keep the hips lifted while rolling the roller away from and toward the body. This exercise strengthens the front and back of the upper legs, hamstrings and quadriceps, as well as the gluteals.

Boat

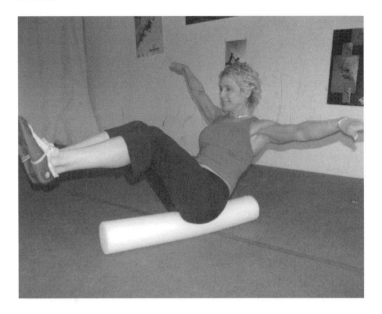

Place the roller vertically on the floor. Sit straddling the roller with one foot on each side. Tighten your stomach and lift your feet off the floor. You can maintain this position with bent knees or straighten the legs for a more advanced exercise. Hold for a count of 20. This exercise strengthens the core and improves balance.

Hyperextension

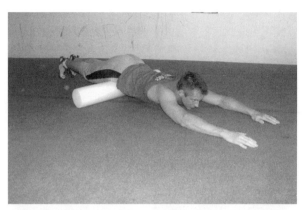

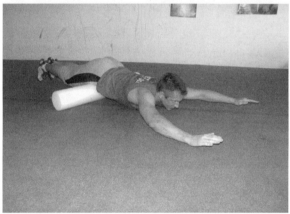

Place the roller horizontally on the floor. Lie on top of the roller with it placed directly above the hips. Straighten your legs and press your toes into the floor. Place your hands out in front like Superman, exhale and lift your chest off the floor. Inhale and lower your chest, releasing the contraction in the back. The exercise strengthens the muscles along the spine and the lower back.

Forward Bend with Calf Stretch

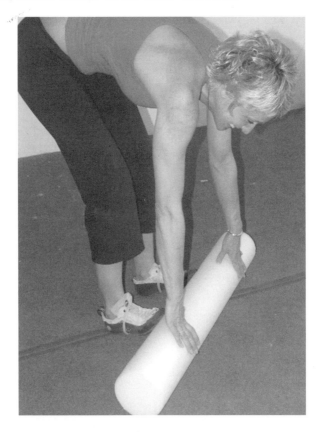

Place the roller horizontally on the floor in front of you. Stand with your toes up on the roller and your heels on the floor. Bend forward from the waist and place your hands on the roller. Hold for a count of 30. This is an intense stretch for the calves, lower back and hamstrings.

Medicine Balls

A medicine ball is a large, heavy, stuffed ball used in conditioning exercises. One prior use of the medicine ball was on marine ships. The marine doctors would prescribe exercises of throwing balls filled with sand in order to alleviate sea sickness symptoms. The use of the medicine ball has resurged in recent years due to its variability and proven results.

Balls provide an alternative to dumbbells. The exercises are not limited by the heavy metal of dumbbells. The soft weighted ball allows for movements that wouldn't be safe with a weighted bar. The types of medicine balls vary from those with bounce to those with no bounce. Some also come with handles or straps on the sides for ease of other movements and to enable a greater variety of movement. For our purposes, a traditional 8-10-pound medicine ball will provide the necessary strength tool.

Push-ups on the Medicine Ball

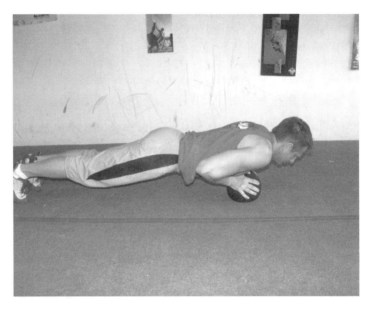

Place the medicine ball on the ground. Kneel behind the ball and place both hands on top of it. Extend the legs straight out behind the body. Inhale, bend your elbows and lower your chest toward the floor. Exhale, straighten the elbows and press back up to the start position. For a more advanced exercise, begin with the medicine ball under one hand. Execute the push-up, and at the top of the movement roll the ball to the other hand. Repeat 2-3 sets of 8-10 repetitions. This exercise strengthens the arms, shoulders, abs, back and chest.

Lunges

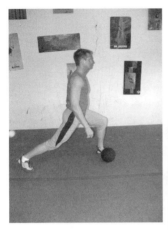

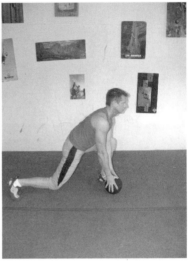

Place the ball on the ground. Stand in a lunge position with the left leg forward and the right leg about two feet behind. Place your left foot next to the medicine ball. Inhale, bend the legs, lower the body toward the floor and reach down to pick up the medicine ball. Exhale and straighten the legs, returning to the starting position. On the next lunge, set the ball down. Repeat 2-3 sets of 8-10 repetitions. This exercise strengthens the legs.

Throw and Catch

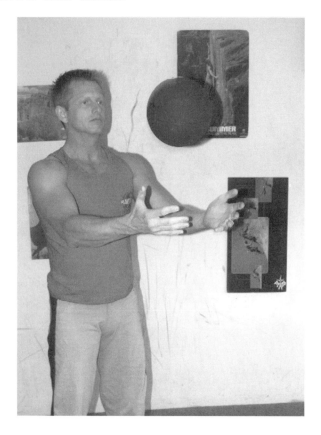

Stand tall and hold the medicine ball in your hands. Place the palms facing up so that the hands are underneath the ball. Tuck your elbows into your rib cage as if you had a belt strapping down your arms. Exhale and throw the ball in the air, keeping the arms in the tucked position. Catch the ball without moving the elbows, but lower the hands toward the hips. Repeat 2-3 sets of 8-10 repetitions. This strengthens the muscles of the upper and lower arms as well as the hands.

Foot Toss

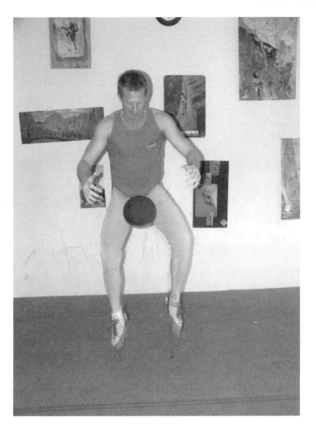

Stand tall with the feet approximately hip-distance apart. Place the medicine ball between your feet on the ground. Exhale and jump up, holding the ball between your feet. Toss the ball into your hands while you're in the air. After you catch the ball, drop it back between your feet. Repeat 2-3 sets of 8-10 repetitions. This exercise strengthens the legs, core and arms, as well as improves mental focus.

Mountain Climbers

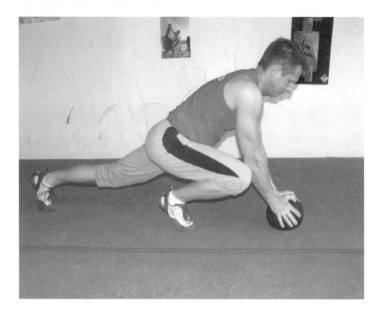

Place the ball on the ground and your hands on the ball. Extend the legs out behind you, keeping the hips off the floor. Exhale and bring your right foot closer to the ball. After a quick touch to the floor, move your right foot back to the starting position. As the right foot moves back, the left foot moves forward. Continue, quickly alternating these foot touches as you hold the abdominal muscles pulled in and the arms stable. Repeat 2-3 sets of 8-10 repetitions. This strengthens the arms, legs and the core.

Sit Back Twists

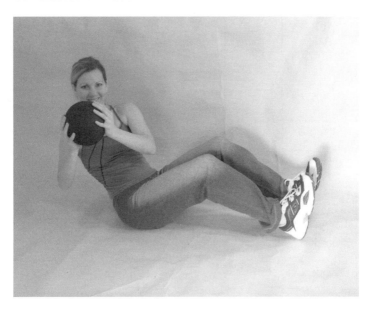

Sit with your knees bent and toes pointed up toward the ceiling. Hold the medicine ball in both hands in front of your chest. Pull your stomach in tight, point your right elbow to the back of the room, inhale and lower your back toward the floor. Exhale and bring your body back to center. Inhale, point your left elbow to the back of the room and lower your back toward the floor at approximately a 45-degree angle. Exhale and release back to center. Repeat 2-3 sets of 8-10 repetitions. This exercise strengthens the abs and back.

For a week of workouts with props, pick one prop per day and work the entire body with that prop. See the following table for an example:

Off the Wall: Exercises for Climbers

Mon.	Tue.	Wed.	Thu.	Fri.
STABILITY BALL WORKOUT Two-Ball Pec Deck Push-ups One-Legged Dead Lift Wall Squat Tricep Lift Oblique Lift	REST or CLIMB	ROLLER WORKOUT Squats Push-ups Bridge Boat Hyperextension Calf Stretch	REST or CLIMB	MEDICINE BALL Push-ups Lunges Throw/ Catch Foot Toss Mountain Climbers Sit-back Twist

Chapter 6

Flexibility, Range of Motion and Mental Focus

Flexibility and Range of Motion

Often a space of two inches can mean the difference in landing a hold or missing it. This lack of reach can be the result of an inflexible muscular system. When the body is tight, it cannot function at its optimal performance level. Fortunately, by spending a little bit of time every week doing flexibility exercises, you can gain that extra two inches and feel confident that you'll be able to climb whatever wall is placed in front of you.

A tight muscle is also a weak muscle. A tight muscle holds the body in a limited range of motion. If we were to move the muscle beyond its range, the muscle could tear. A flexible joint requires less energy to move through its full range of motion. That means more energy to climb higher. By keeping the joints and muscles flexible, the muscle is strong throughout its entire range. Flexibility training also trains the mind to be more in tune with the muscles, so the muscles respond faster to climbing demands.

Before you climb, stretching can improve your reach, aid in the dynamic moves and decrease your risk of injury to the joints and muscles. After climbing, stretching can realign any muscular imbalances that resulted from the climb. Climbing does not use each muscle group the same way and these imbalances can lead to soreness and pain. A simple stretching routine can help to alleviate aches, improve circulation to the joints, and

ease the muscle back into normal resting length, returning the body to good posture.

Overstretching can lead to joint instability. That is why
the need exists for a well-rounded program of strength,
flexibility and relaxation.

How To's of Stretching

- Stretch a muscle when it's warm. After a brief 5-10
  minute warm-up of walking, bouldering or traversing, the muscles will stretch better.
- Stretch the muscle groups one at a time.
- The stretches are to be slow and controlled. Hold
  for 15-30 seconds.
- Do not bounce.
- Stretch to the point of feeling resistance, but not to
  the point of pain.
- For maximum benefit, 3-5 repetitions of each
  stretch should be completed.
- For range-of-motion improvement, daily participation in stretching is recommended.

The following is a collection of "on-the-wall stretches,"
exercises that can be performed wherever there is a wall
and some free space.

Frog Stretch

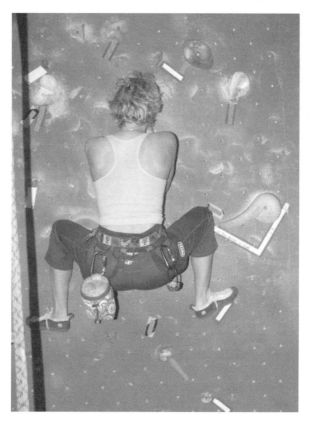

Place your feet on two holds that are close together and slightly wider than shoulder-width apart. Bend your knees out to the sides, lowering the hips toward the feet. Grab onto any hand holds and press your hips toward the wall. This stretch helps your ability to bring your weight in toward the wall when climbing. Hold this stretch for a count of 15-30 seconds.

Split Stretch

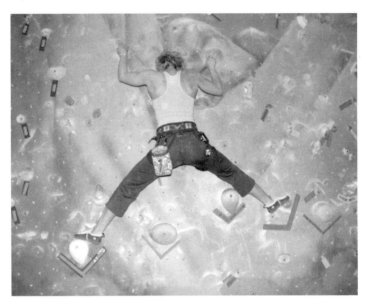

This stretch works best in a corner of a wall. Place your feet as far apart as is comfortable on two different walls. Grab hand holds over the right leg and press your chest and hips toward the wall. Hold for a count of 15-30 seconds, then walk your hands over the left leg. Hold for a count of 15-30 seconds.

Groin Stretch

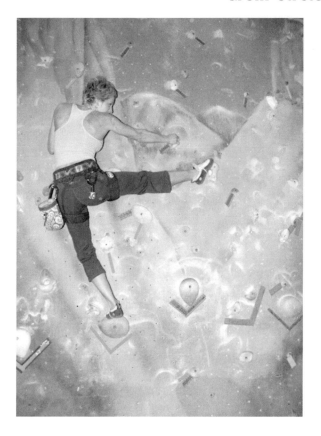

Place your left foot on the wall directly underneath the body. Raise your right leg to a hold near shoulder height. Grasp any hand holds in front of you and press your hips into the wall. Hold for a count of 15-30 seconds. Repeat with the right leg underneath and the left leg raised.

The exercises on the following pages are forearm stretches to be performed between climbs.

Prayer Hands Up and Down

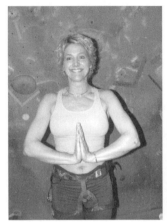

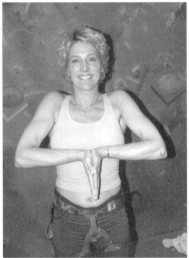

Place the palms of the hands together in front of the body. With the fingers facing up, gently lower the hands toward the floor. Keep the palms pressing against each other. Hold for a count of 15-30 seconds. Next, keep the palms pressing together and turn the fingers toward the floor. Raise the palms toward the ceiling and hold for a count of 15-30.

Mr. Magoo

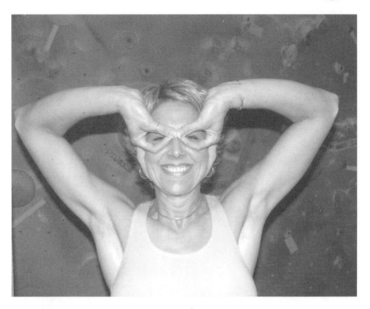

Make circles with the hands by placing the thumb and the index fingers together. Place the remaining three fingers on the sides of the face with the fingertips pointing down. Bring the circles up in front of the eyes, as if they were glasses. Hold for a count of 15-30 seconds.

The exercises on the following pages are after-climbing stretches that can be performed at any time needed.

Shoulder Stretch

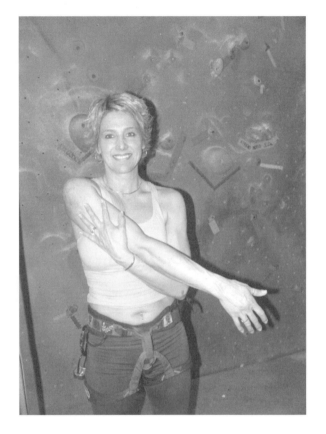

Reach the right arm straight across your body. Place the left hand on the back of the right arm and apply gentle pressure, pulling on the shoulder. Hold for 15-30 seconds and repeat on the left arm.

Tricep Stretch

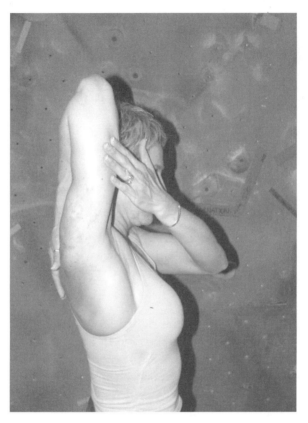

Point the right elbow toward the ceiling and place the right hand between your shoulder blades. Place the left hand on the back of the right arm and apply gentle pressure to stretch the back of the arm. Hold for 15-30 seconds and repeat with the left arm.

Hamstring Stretch

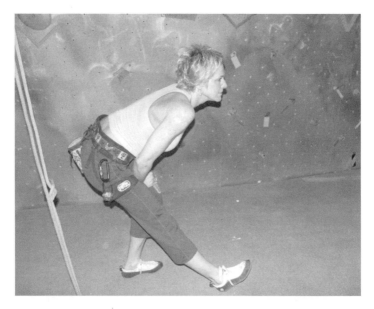

Standing tall, extend the right foot out onto the floor. Place the right heel into the floor and bend the left leg. Place your hands on your left leg, and sink your chest toward your legs. Keep your head up and look forward while holding the stretch. Hold for 15-30 seconds and repeat on the opposite leg.

Quadriceps Stretch

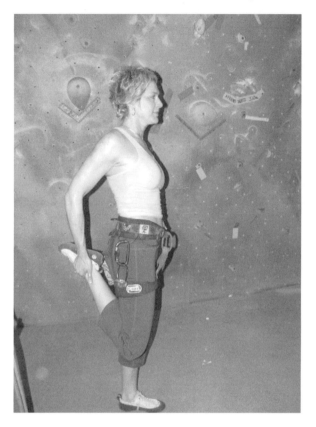

Standing tall, shift your weight onto your left leg. Bend your right leg, bringing your foot behind you. Reach back with your right hand to grasp your right ankle. Hold for a count of 15-30 seconds, then release and repeat on the opposite leg.

Hip Stretch

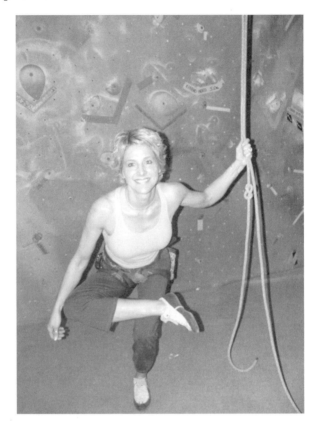

After the quadriceps stretch, bring your right foot to rest on the front of the left leg above the left knee. Gently bend the left knee until you feel the stretch in your right hip. You can also apply gentle pressure to the top of the right leg, pressing the knee in the direction of the floor. Hold for 15-30 seconds and repeat on the opposite leg.

Chest Stretch

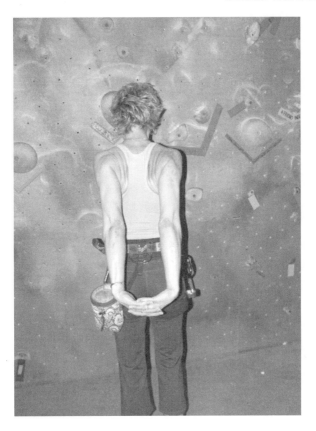

Standing tall, lace your hands behind your back, palms up. Keep your arms and back straight as you lift your arms as high as possible. Do not bend into the stretch. Hold for a count of 15-30 seconds.

The exercises on the following pages are hand, wrist and finger stretches, for use at any time.

Thumb Stretch

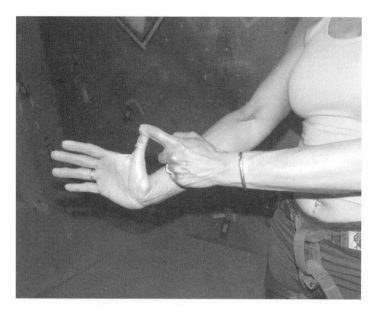

Extend your right arm out in front of your body. Keep the palm facing toward the center as if shaking someone's hand. Grasp your right thumb with your left hand and gently pull the thumb toward the body. Hold for a count of 15-30 seconds and repeat on the left hand.

Finger Stretches

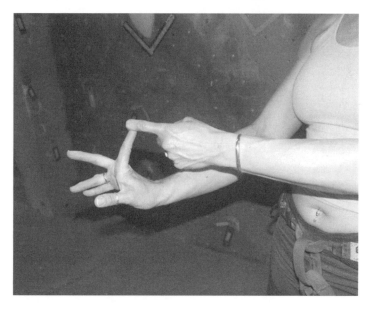

Gently pull back on the index finger of the right hand with the left hand. Carefully work through each finger, pulling it toward the body and pushing it away. Apply even pressure on each finger and do not tug the joint. Repeat the entire sequence three times.

Figure Eights

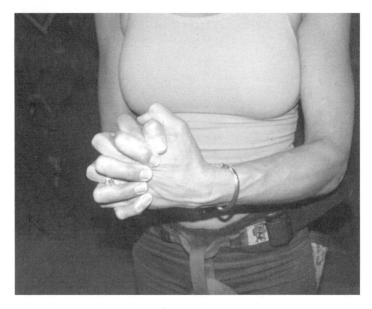

Clasp the hands together in front of the body. Interlace the fingers and rest them on the opposite hand. Bend the elbows. Rotate your hands in a figure eight. Rotate 8-10 times for two sets.

Mental Focus

Focusing the mind is simply paying attention. On the wall, if you begin to think about work or other responsibilities, your focus will be disrupted. By using proper concentration when climbing, you'll be able to reach greater heights than ever before. A climbing wall is like a puzzle. A certain sequence of hand and foot holds needs to be followed to reach the top of the climb. When concentration is interrupted, the climb can be unsuccessful.

Mental focus allows for fluid movement on the wall. Having control over the body and mind leads to more talented climbing. When you are focused, technique gets stronger and each move becomes more specific and confident. But when focus is scattered, the body is taxed due to the extra time hanging on the wall trying to determine the next sequence. Plan your sequence before you place one hand or foot on the wall. Think ahead of the wall right in front of you and try to imagine hanging from the wall in various positions. Look also for places to rest on the wall, where you can plan your next series of moves. All of this takes focus and concentration.

You may find that on some days it's easier to map the route up the wall. You feel in tune and focused. On other days, no matter what you try, you can't seem to see the series on the wall. Mental concentration can be improved with exercise. The mind is like a muscle and the more you train and strengthen it, the better it will perform for you.

Successful mind focus can begin during a training program. It is important to concentrate in the moment and be mindful of every repetition. Being mindful means working out with an inward focus of concentration. It doesn't mean lifting the heaviest weight or completing the most repetitions. The focus is on the movement it-self, the range of motion and breath control.

It is also good to add here that this reduces competition. When working out or climbing, your competition should be with only yourself. Do not compare yourself to what others are doing. If you're inwardly focusing, you won't notice when others lift more or climb higher. You'll be paying attention to your own personal gains, and that's all that matters.

Along with mindfulness comes visual imagery. When you stand at the bottom of a climb, your own perceptions of that climb will have an effect on the outcome. While looking up the wall, "see" yourself at the top of the climb. It is important to visualize the results you want to see. Your brain only knows what you tell it, so be mindful of the messages you send.

Yoga exercise is a tool to build mental focus. The yoga poses use specific body alignments and a breathing style that clears the mind. Eventually, this clearing of the mind becomes natural and carries over onto the wall. The climber who has developed a quiet mind will focus on the task at hand and block out any distractions such as noise, music or discomfort.

The following exercises are helpful for climber's bod-ies and minds:

Spinal Balance

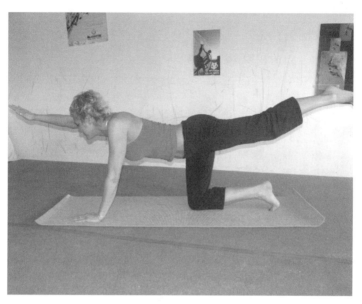

Kneel on all fours with your knees under your hips and your hands under your shoulders. Inhale and extend the right arm and left leg. Keep the arm and leg in line with the body. Tighten the stomach and hold the spine straight. Concentrate on reaching away from your body through your fingers and toes. Exhale and release. Inhale and repeat with the left arm and right leg. This exercise helps coordinate between the opposite sides of your body. Complete 8-10 repetitions on each side.

Downward-Facing Dog

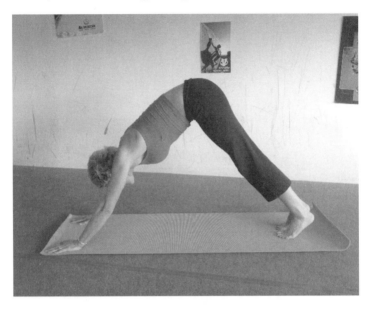

Remain kneeling, then straighten your legs and press your hips toward the ceiling. You will look as if you're an inverted letter V. The arms and legs are straight and your heels are pressing toward the floor. Relax your neck by shaking your head "no" and focusing on your feet. This exercise stretches forearms, wrists, calves, upper back and shoulders. Hold for 5-10 breaths.

Side Straddle

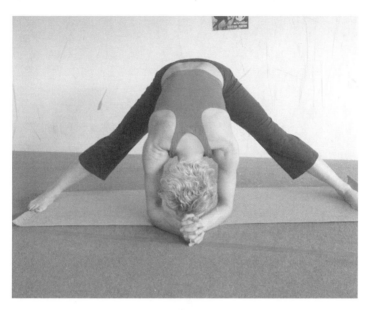

Stand with your legs straight and your feet approximately 3-4 feet apart. Bend forward from your waist and place your hands on the floor, allowing your head to drop down. If you're feeling comfortable, come all the way down onto your elbows. Slightly bend the knees if you feel any discomfort in the back. This exercise stretches the groin area, inner thighs and the hamstrings. Hold for 5-10 breaths.

Tree

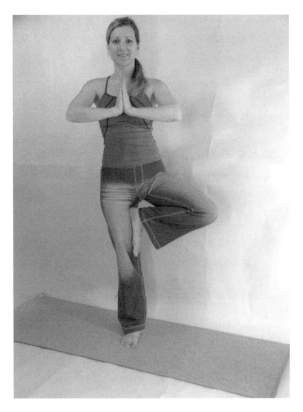

Standing tall, shift the weight of your body onto your right leg. Place the left foot next to the right ankle, calf, or inner thigh. Avoid placing it right on the knee. Find a focal point to concentrate on as you bring your hands together in front of the body. When comfortable, extend straight arms overhead as if they are branches of a tree. Hold for 5-10 breaths and repeat on the left leg. The tree pose brings balance, strengthens the legs and stretches the inner thigh and back.

Warrior II

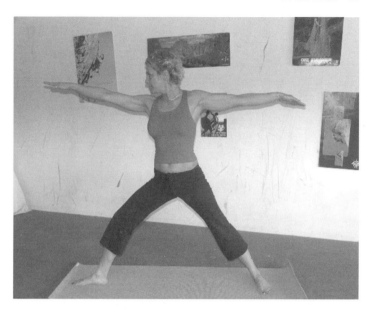

Step into a lunge position with the right leg in front and the left leg behind. Place the heel of the left foot onto the floor and align the arch of that left foot with the heel of the right foot. Open the hips and extend the arms out at shoulder height with the right arm

over the right leg and the left arm over the left leg. Pull your shoulders down away from your ears. Focus on your right middle finger. Bend your right knee to a 90-degree angle with the knee remaining over the heel. Hold for 5-10 breaths and repeat on the left leg. Warrior II strengthens the legs and stretches the chest and inner thighs.

Reverse Warrior

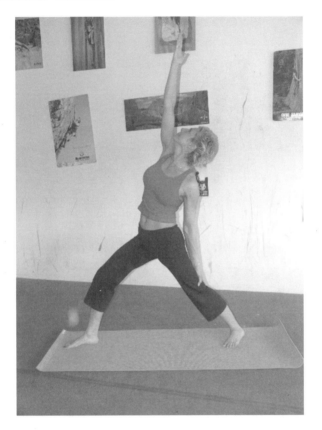

From the Warrior II position, slowly lower the left hand down the left leg, raising the straight right arm toward the ceiling. Look up to the right hand. Keep the right knee bent and drop the left hand as far as comfortable down the left leg. Hold for 5-10 breaths and repeat on the left leg. This exercise aids in balance, strengthens the legs, and stretches the waist, inner thighs and back.

Crane

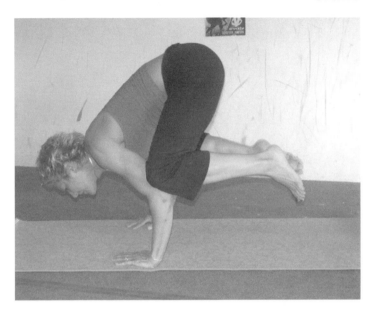

Stand tall with your feet hip-distance apart. Bend forward from the waist and place your hands on the floor slightly wider than shoulder-distance apart. Bend your knees and your elbows, and rest your knees on the backs of your arms. Begin by lifting one foot off the floor at a time, then advance to balancing on the hands. Your focus is straight down to the floor. Hold for 5-10 breaths. The crane pose strengthens the upper body and the core.

Bow

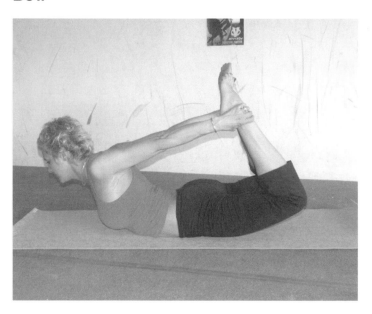

Lie down on your stomach. Bend your right knee and reach back with the right hand for the right ankle. Bend your left knee and reach back with the left hand for the left ankle. Exhale and lift your chest, arms and legs toward the ceiling. Look straight ahead and concentrate on the breath. This is a great stretch for climbers, as it opens the front of the body and strengthens the back.

Corpse

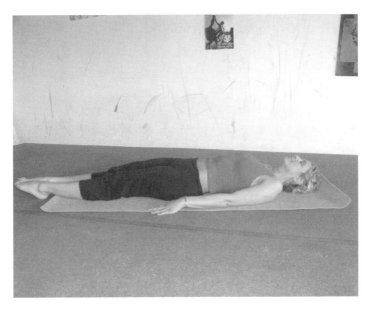

Lie down on your back. Rest your arms along your sides with your palms facing up. Allow your shoulders and ankles to rest on the floor. Close your eyes and focus on your breathing for five minutes. Practice in a room where there are no distractions. If you feel your mind wandering, bring the focus back to the breath. This is good practice for focusing solely on the wall. The more practice we have with quieting everything around us, the easier it is to get into the focused frame of mind.

Adding a few yoga poses to your weekly strengthening workout will improve your flexibility and mental focus. The following table shows an example of how to combine exercises:

Off the Wall: Exercises for Climbers

Mon.	Tue.	Wed.	Thu.	Fri.
Spinal Balance Down Dog Side Straddle	REST or CLIMB Hand and Finger Stretches	Warrior II Reverse Warrior Tree	REST or CLIMB Wrist and Forearm Stretches	Crane Bow Corpse

Chapter 7
Cardiovascular Training

The cardiovascular (CV) system includes the heart, lungs, blood vessels and blood stream. When these are functioning at peak performance, we feel great. The body is getting the oxygen it needs in order to survive.

We can keep this system strong by participating in cardio exercise 30-45 minutes, 3-5 days a week. This may sound like a lot of time, but knowing that a healthy CV system reduces the risk of heart attacks, strokes, high blood pressure, high cholesterol and being over-weight should be enough to begin a training program.

For climbing, cardiovascular strength is necessary to bring oxygen into all of the muscle systems. It also helps when climbing for speed. The heart will keep the oxygen flowing, allowing you to race to the top of the wall.

Your CV system is used specifically for longer climbs with easier holds. Training the CV system increases the capillary network to encourage more efficient oxygen delivery to the muscles and waste removal from the muscles. That burning sensation you feel in the muscles while climbing is the result of a build-up of lactic acid in the muscle tissue. On the longer climbs, the body's CV system works with oxygen to remove this lactic acid from the muscles, allowing you to continue the climb.

Moreover, *The British Journal of Sports Medicine* in September of 1997 published data indicating "that indoor rock climbing is a good activity to increase cardiorespiratory fitness and muscular endurance." So whether training for climbing or climbing for health, indoor rock climbing brings the best of aerobic and anaerobic workouts into one.

A training effect will occur if all of the principles of **FITT** are adopted. FITT stands for Frequency, Intensity, Time and Type.

Frequency is how often an exercise is performed. A minimum of three days per week of CV exercise is needed to see improvements. Less than three days and the body maintains, but will not improve, its CV system.

Intensity of a CV exercise is based on the correct heart rate range. For target heart rate range, we use the following formula: (220-age) x .6 = low range, (220-age) x .85 = high range. For example, a 30-year-old's heart rate range will be: 220 - 30= 190, 190 x .6 = 114 for the low range, and for the high range 220 - 30=190, 190 x .85 = 161.

When the heart rate falls below 60%, the body receives minimal cardiovascular benefits. If the heart rate increases too much over 85% the body burns sugar as its energy source instead of fat. Between 60-85% the body improves cardiovascular health and burns fat as the fuel.

Time spent in CV exercise should be between 30 and 45 minutes. This means that your heart rate will be elevated for that amount of time.

Types of CV exercise include walking, jogging, running, swimming, cycling, roller blading, treadmill climbing, etc. These are exercises that elevate the heart rate and use oxygen. These are full-body exercises.

CV exercises should be preceded by a warm-up. These 3-4 minutes prior to a workout should consist of a similar exercise, but at a lower intensity. You gradually want to increase the heart rate into the training zone, instead of jumping right into it. This gives the body time to adjust to the activity and allows the CV system to work most efficiently. You can avoid injuries this way. The exercises should be smooth, controlled and use as much of the body as possible.

CV exercises need to be followed by a cool-down. Quickly stopping an exercise can cause the blood to pool in the legs which could lead to passing out. Like the warm-up, the cool down is 3-4 minutes of less intense exercise to bring the heart rate back to pre-exercise levels.

As you can see, the heart rate is the key for CV training. The following table gives a brief overview of heart rate ranges in a 10-second count. For more detailed numbers, use the above formula.

10-Second Heart Rate Count			
AGE	60%	70%	85%
20-22	20	23	28
23-25	19	23	28
26-31	19	22	27
32-34	19	21	26
35-43	18	21	26
44-46	17	20	25
47-52	17	20	24
53-55	17	19	23
56-60	16	19	23
61-70	15	18	22
71-75	14	16	20

When the heart rate is lower than the chart, the benefits will not be as great. When the heart rate is higher than the chart, you've gone into exercising without as much oxygen. When strength training, your heart rate will rise into this level. That's acceptable, because you only participate in the exercise for 30 seconds to a minute, then you take a rest to allow the heart rate to recover before proceeding with the next exercise.

For CV health, the goal is to keep the heart rate elevated into the correct range for 30-45 minutes. Take your pulse approximately 15 minutes into a workout to determine if you're in the correct range. You then can adjust your intensity according to your heart rate.

To find the heart rate, use the first two fingers. The thumb has a pulse of its own, so don't use it. Place the two fingers gently on the side of the neck, just above the collar bone to find the carotid pulse. Do not apply too much pressure here. You can also find the radial pulse in the wrist by placing the two fingers on the underside of the wrist.

Using the palpitation at either place, count the beats that you feel in 10 seconds. You can also take your pulse for 15 seconds and multiply it by four to find your beats per minute. Try to keep your feet moving while taking your pulse so the heart rate doesn't slow and the blood doesn't pool in the legs.

Find your age and heart rate number on the table on the previous page, or multiply the 10-second count number by six and check your personal formula. We want that number to be in the 60-85% range, or somewhere on the above chart.

The following table shows an example of a week with CV exercise. This is in addition to any strength training for that week.

Mon.	Tue.	Wed.	Thu.	Fri.
Walk for 45 minutes	REST or CLIMB	Cycle for 45 minutes	REST or CLIMB	Swim for 45 min. (Swimming heart rate is 10-13 beats below heart rate range for land exercise.)

Chapter 8
Plyometric Training

Plyometric exercises (plyos) have their roots in jump-training exercises. Plyometrics means "measurable increases." *Measurable* increases. Especially in your dynamic moves, these jump-training exercises will bring you more explosive power. A dynamic move, or dyno, is a movement where you cannot simply reach out for a hand hold. It's a hold that you need to leave the wall for a second in order to reach. The legs propel you up as you jump toward that higher hold. Practicing plyometrics will also strengthen the joints of the lower body to protect you when falling or when landing after being belayed.

Plyos link strength with speed of movement to produce power. The exercises begin with the muscles in a slightly elongated or stretched position. The muscles do not stay here long because they quickly move into a shortening contraction. When you repeatedly train muscles this way, the result is a more forceful movement for propelling the body. The muscles, tendons and nerve receptors increase their sensitivity to the movements and respond with increased power.

To get an idea of the movement, imagine that the ground is a big spring. Stand on this spring and propel yourself up. When you land, you do not stay because are immediately propelled up again.

Do plyometric exercises work for already-trained athletes? A study performed on 26 athletic men over the course of eight weeks looked at the difference between heavy- and light-loaded jump squats on various performance levels. The results are found in the *Journal of Strength and Conditioning Research*, February 2002. The study concluded that training with light-loaded jump squats results in increased movement capabilities.

Do plyometric exercises work for women? In general, women have weaker leg strength than men. Also, the positioning of wider hips puts extra strain on the knee joint. An article presented in *Athletic Therapy Today*, July 2001, suggests that core and leg-strength exercises should be a focus in a woman's injury-prevention or rehabilitative program. It suggests that agility and landing (jump-training) exercises should also be a focus in this program.

Do plyometric exercises work for children? Another study in the *Journal of Sports Medicine and Physical Fitness*, June 2001, looked at the effects of plyometric training on elite junior basketball players. This study concluded that even with a limited amount of plyometric training, jumping performance could improve in elite junior basketball players.

Research has shown that plyometric exercises are effective. Plyos work well for trained athletes and the average male or female. Dynamic power will be increased by adding a plyometric workout to your training routine.

Keep in mind that plyos are not designed to increase aerobic capacity or strengthen the cardiovascular system, so the body needs a complete rest (45-60 seconds) between each set of exercises. Plyos can be added to a training program once or twice a week with at least one day of rest between training. Plyos are not to be used as the sole form of training. Your workout program must include cardiovascular exercise and strength training topped off with plyos to bring the explosive power.

As with any training program, plyo workouts should begin with a warm-up. A warm-up can be a smaller version of the exercises you will be performing — a short walk, a march in place, a quick bike ride, or anything that moves the entire body in a full range of motion for approximately five minutes.

Throughout the workout, feet should be nearly flat in all landings. The ball of the foot may touch first, but the rest of the foot should quickly follow. The arms help to force the body into the ground by beginning behind the midline of the body and then swinging rapidly forward and up for liftoff. Total time spent in plyometric exercises should not exceed 20 to 30 minutes.

The following exercises will develop strength in the legs, the core and the arms. With consistent use of these exercises, you will see noticeable results in your climbing and dynamic bouldering moves. Begin with one set of 10-15 repetitions and increase to three sets of 10-15 repetitions for each exercise. Correct form is the most important element. And remember to breathe!

Some of the exercises use a medicine ball for additional variety and intensity.

Tuck Jumps

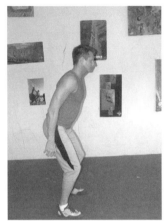

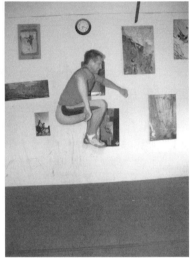

Stand with your feet shoulder-distance apart and knees slightly bent. Begin with your arms behind your body. Use the arms to help you jump up and bring your knees to your chest. As you land, immediately jump up again, keeping ground contact time to a minimum.

Squat Depth Jump

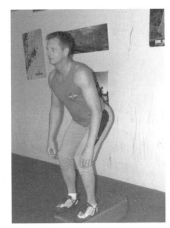

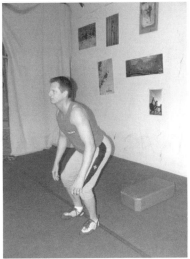

Stand on a box with your knees bent into a half squat. Place your toes close to the edge. Step off the box and land in a 90-degree squat position. Jump up out of this squat and land in another squat. Return back to the box and repeat.

Trunk Rotation

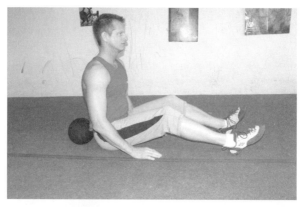

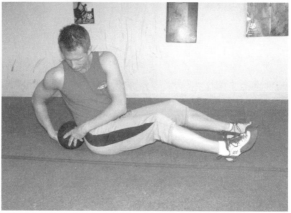

Sit on the floor with your legs spread. Place a medicine ball behind your back. Rotate to the right, pick up the ball, bring it around to your left side and replace it behind your back. Repeat 10-15 times and then reverse.

Medicine Ball Grab

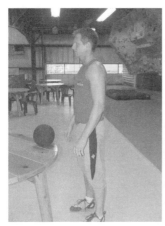

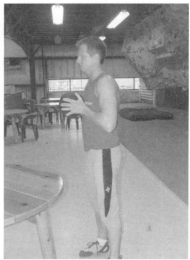

Place your medicine ball on a box in front of you. The box should be slightly lower than hip level. Stand facing the ball with your knees slightly bent. Quickly reach forward, grab the ball and bring it into your chest. Then just as quickly release it back down. Repeat the exercise 10 to 15 times.

Incline Push-up Depth Jump

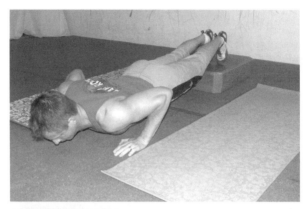

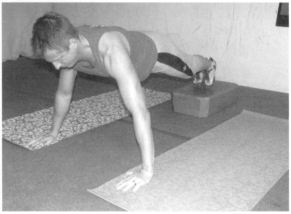

Place two exercise mats on the floor approximately two feet apart. Place a box at the end of the mats. Begin with your feet on the box and your hands on the floor between the two mats. Start in a push-up position, with your elbows slightly bent. Push up off the ground with your hands and land with one hand on each mat. Push up off the mats, and catch yourself in the starting position.

Clap Push-ups

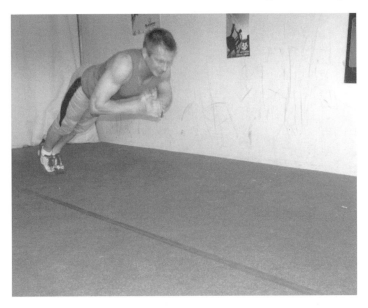

Begin in a push-up position. Bend your elbows, lowering your chest toward the floor. Straighten your arms and, at the top of the movement, lift your hands off the floor and clap them together. Land with your arms in a lowered push-up position. Straighten your arms and repeat the clap.

Planks with Foot Jump

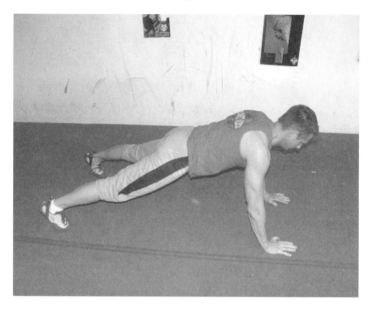

Place your hands on the floor approximately shoulder-distance apart. Straighten your legs behind your body and rest your toes on the floor. Press your hips toward the floor, keeping your body in a straight line. Jump your feet apart, maintaining the plank position. Without resting, quickly jump the feet back together.

Plyo Pull-ups

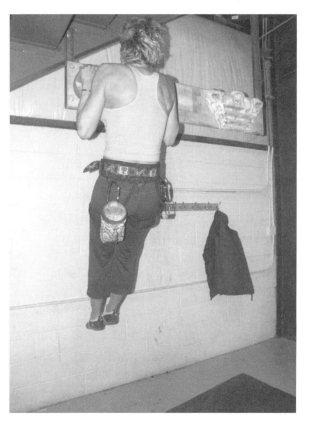

Hold onto a bar with your hands wider than shoulder-distance apart. Bend your elbows and pull your chin up over the bar. Let go of the bar, straighten your arms and catch the bar with your hands at the bottom of the movement. Pull yourself back up, release and begin again.

Campus Board Drills

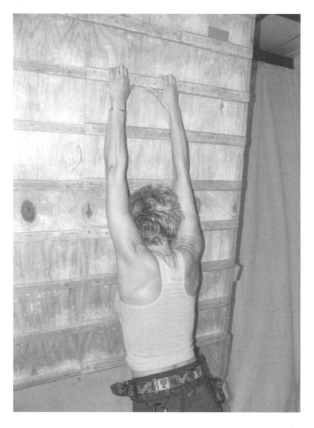

A campus board is a wooden board with fingertip rungs spaced at different intervals. There are no feet involved with the use of a campus board. A campus board is one of the best training tools for increasing fingertip strength. These can be found at indoor climbing gyms or you can make your own.

Begin with both hands on a high rung. Let go and drop to catch yourself on a lower rung. Immediately propel yourself up to a higher rung. Repeat until fatigued.

Follow the plyometric exercises with a cool-down and some stretching time. Take a few minutes to walk around, gathering your breath and relaxing the trained muscles. Sit on the floor, straighten your legs out in front of you and fold the upper body over the legs, bringing the hands down the legs to a comfortable position. This will stretch the backs of the legs and lower back. Next, lie down on your back and pull both knees into the chest to stretch the lower back. Roll over onto your stomach, bend the right knee, reach back with the right hand and grasp the right ankle to stretch the front of the right leg. Repeat on the left leg. Each stretch is held for 30-45 seconds. These are static stretches, so do not bounce.

The following table shows an example of how to split up the plyometric exercises into a weekly routine.

Mon.	Tue.	Wed.	Thu.	Fri.
Squat Depth Jumps Planks with Jump Feet Campus Board Drills	REST or CLIMB	Tuck Jumps Incline Push-ups Depth Jumps Medicine Ball Grab	REST or CLIMB	Plyo Pull-ups Clap Push-ups Trunk Rotation

Chapter 9
Circuit Training

Circuit training is a type of interval training that provides a total body workout in a quick amount of time. Another benefit is that it erases the boredom that often comes from indoor exercises because the workouts are constantly changing. Every day the workout can be different, yet still provide the strengthening and overall body health benefits you're seeking.

Circuit training is based on a set amount of time spent in different activities. It alternates bursts of intense activity with less intense activity. The workout consists of small stations, alternating a cardiovascular exercise with a strengthening exercise. Once or twice through all the stations completes the circuit. The total time spent in each station can vary, but 1½ minutes in each works well. The workout can last anywhere from 20 to 60 minutes depending on the needs of the day. This workout should be performed with a day of rest between to allow muscles recovery time.

Not only is circuit training an efficient workout style, it also helps to avoid injuries that come from repetitive activities and overuse. Since the exercise stations are changed every day, the body is allowed to work through the different planes and ranges of motion. This protects the joints and muscles as well as strengthens them in various positions. Circuit training maintains the heart rate at an increased level to allow for aerobic conditioning throughout the entire workout. Even during the strengthening exercises, the heart rate will not recover to the resting rate. This constant elevation requires the body to use fat as the energy source, leading to reduced weight levels and lower body fat percentages.

The strength gained through the workout increases muscle tissue in the body. In turn, the increased muscle tissue increases the body's metabolism. Muscle tissue burns more calories in a day than fat tissue, so your body uses the food you eat as energy to maintain lean body mass as opposed to storing the food intake as fat.

Another benefit of circuit training is that it can be performed solely by using the body in various positions. There is no need for a lot of equipment or large, costly exercise machines. It can be practiced anywhere, indoors or out. However, there are some recommendations for an indoor, at-home workout. You'll need a stopwatch, timer or clock to keep track of the time in each station; a small space in which to move around and not be compromised; and dumbbells, benches, balls and mats for the various stations. You should set up the exercise stations prior to beginning the workout.

Basic Circuit Training

The basic circuit training workout uses set intervals of 1½ minutes, alternating an aerobic exercise with a strength training exercise. There is no rest between stations. You move quickly from one station to the next, so it's wise to have the exercises written down, placed in order and have the necessary equipment available.

You will need to choose five cardiovascular exercises, such as walking, jogging, jump rope, hopping and stair climbing. You will alternate these exercises with strength exercises. Examples of strength exercises are located throughout this book. The most readily available are squats, push-ups, dips, lunges and pull-ups.

Begin with a warm-up of 3-4 minutes of walking.

Then get your stopwatch ready and walk for 1½ minutes. Next you will squat for 1½ minutes. The sequence continues with jogging, push-ups, jumping rope, dips, hopping, lunges, stair climbing and pull-ups. Repeat this sequence of exercises 2-3 times for maximum benefit.

You can vary the time spent in each station. You can also change the order of the stations, so that two CV exercises are followed by one strength exercise, or two strength exercises are followed by a CV exercise. Circuits can be set up based on your particular needs that day. Using the plyometric exercises we learned, you can alternate a plyo exercise with a regular strength exercise. For example, follow a tuck jump with a push-up or a trunk rotation with a squat.

Circuit training can also be taken on the wall for advanced training. These circuits can be based on time or on a set number of moves. For example, climb for one minute, then hang for 30 seconds. Continue alternating climbing and hanging until you've reached the top. This works particularly well when traversing an indoor wall.

You can also execute a climbing circuit by climbing for 10 moves then resting for one minute, climbing for 10 moves then resting for one minute. A partner can help keep the time and help you count the moves.

Either of these styles of circuits will help build endurance on the wall. By using the circuit training, you're not climbing at top level and your fingers and grip will not completely burn out on every climb. You'll train the muscles to work hard and then recover. This allows for toxin removal and the ability to climb for a longer period of time. It is not recommended to climb this way on every climb, as there are days you'll want to tax your muscles and make it to the top as quickly as possible.

The following table shows examples of circuit training workouts. The sequences are to be repeated 2-3 times depending on the strength of the day.

Monday	Tuesday	Wednesday	Thursday	Friday
Basic Circuit	*Climbing Circuit*	*Strength Circuit*	*Plyo Circuit*	*Climbing Circuit*
Walk Squat Jog Push-ups Jump Rope Dips Hop Lunges Stair Climbs Pull-ups	1 minute of climb 30 seconds rest 1 minute of climb 30 seconds rest continue until top	Squat Dip Walk Push-ups Abs Jump Rope Pull-ups Lunges Jog	Tuck Jump Push-up Trunk Rotation Squat Ball Grab Lunges Planks Pull-ups Clap-ups Dips	10 moves Rest 10 moves Rest continue until top of the climb

Chapter 10
Training Between Climbs

The time spent between climbs at the climbing gym or outside at the rock can be used to further strengthen and improve the body. Most of us spend "down" time relaxing, eating, resting and talking with our companions. That isn't wasted time, but you can also use this time for yourself. How you spend the time between climbs is also beneficial for recovery. A study published in the *International Journal of Sports Medicine* in April of 2000 found that climbers who used an exercise bike for active recovery after a climb significantly reduced the amount of accumulated blood lactate (lactic acid) within 20 minutes of a difficult climb. Their lactate levels had returned to pre-climb levels. In another group who had passive recovery, the lactate levels remained elevated 30 minutes after climbing. The lactic acid level is what causes the burning sensation in the muscles while climbing, particularly in the forearms. If you can use this in-between time to help remove the lactic acid levels, you encourage repair in the muscles and will be strong again for the next climb.

All it takes is walking around the gym or outside. Walk at a quick pace in order to increase the heart rate to your training level (see the table in Chapter 7). Within 20 minutes you should feel the burning sensation easing and be ready for your next climb.

Everything you need for a complete body workout between climbs can be found at the base. Keep these guidelines in mind:

- Abdominal muscles should be held in tight
- Exhale on the exertion portion of the movement
- Maintain spinal alignment
- Bend the knees slightly while standing
- Complete 2-3 sets of 8-12 repetitions
- Use slow and controlled movements

Pull-ups

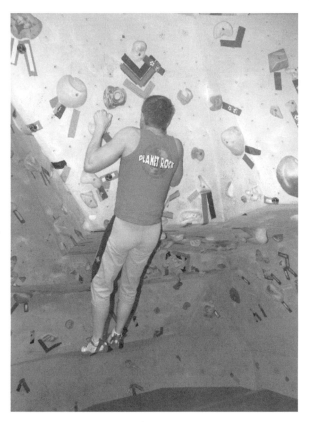

Place your hands on holds or a tree branch slightly wider than shoulder-distance apart with your palms facing away from your body. Bend your elbows, pulling them into your sides as you exhale and lift your chin up over the bar. Inhale, straightening the arms, and slowly release to the start position. This strengthens the back and the arms.

Hanging Knees/Leg Raises

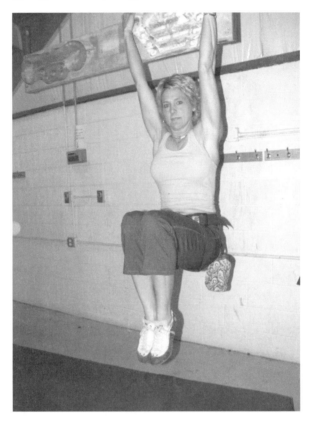

Holding onto a branch or a bar, place your hands shoulder-distance apart with your palms facing away from your body. Straighten your legs underneath you. Keeping your back straight, exhale and pull the knees up into the chest. For an advanced variation, pull your straight legs up to the level of the hips. Inhale and release to start. This strengthens the abdominal muscles.

Wall Push-ups

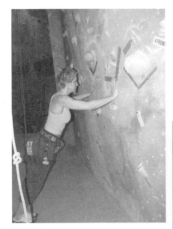

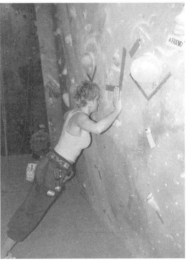

Stand facing a wall. Place your hands on the wall shoulder distance apart. Walk your feet away from the wall so that the body is at a slight angle. The farther the feet are from the wall, the more challenging the exercise will be. Inhale, bend the elbows and bring the chest toward the wall. Exhale, straighten the arms and release to start. For a variation, lift one foot for the first set and the other for the next. This can also be done one arm at a time. This strengthens the chest, arms and core.

Dips

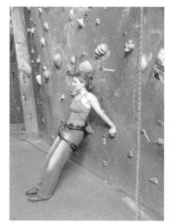

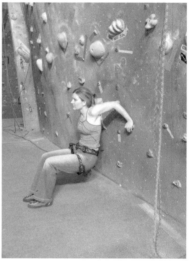

Sit on the side of a large rock, on stairs or in a chair. Place your palms next to your hips. Walk your feet away from the base, leaving your hips suspended in the air. Inhale and bend your elbows behind the body until at a 90-degree angle, lowering your hips toward the ground. Exhale and straighten the arms, raising the hips. For increased intensity, straighten the legs or lift one leg toward the sky. This strengthens the triceps, the back of the upper arm.

Uneven Squats

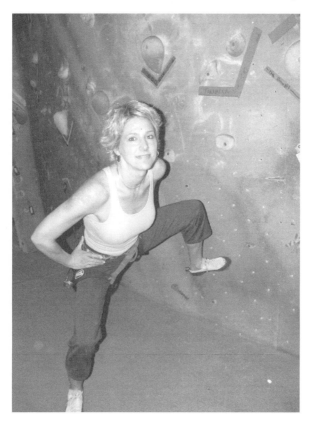

Place one foot on the ground and the other slightly elevated on a rock or wall hold. Align the knees so they are each pointing out over the toes. Inhale and lower the hips until knees are bent at a 90-degree angle. Exhale, straighten the legs and release to start. Do one set with the right leg elevated and one set with the left leg elevated. This exercise strengthens the legs.

Chapter 11
Special Considerations

As previously discussed, rock climbing can lead to finger, hand and wrist injuries. If you do suffer an injury, take time off from climbing and strength training the upper body until that injury heals. You'll want to get back to climbing quickly, and further activity can only prolong the injury.

If you suffer from any back problems, use the suggestions in Chapter 4 to help ease your discomfort. When strength training, always keep your knees slightly bent and do not hyperextend the back. Be especially careful when belaying your partner. Stand farther away from the wall, so that you do not have to look up so dramatically. This will help protect your neck and your spine from further discomfort.

If you have high blood pressure, choose a lighter resistance weight for strength training. Pay particular attention to the breathing guidelines and never hold your breath.

For those with lower body injuries, again, take time off to allow the body to repair. Be careful when landing from a climb and remind your partner to set you down gently. It's helpful to wrap the injured area with a support bandage for additional protection while climbing or training.

If you are pregnant, please check with your doctor before beginning any exercise program. Do not lie on your back for exercises after the fourth month. As a general guideline, your heart rate should not exceed 140 beats per minute when participating in cardiovascular exercise.

Diabetics should follow their doctor's advice for an exercise program. Keep a snack on hand and monitor your glucose levels.

Off-the-Wall Reminders

- Choose a weight amount that challenges the last two repetitions of each exercise.
- Follow your heart rate range guidelines during cardiovascular exercise.
- Use a full range of motion when strength training. Avoid locking the joints.
- Use a complete exhale and inhale for each movement. This will slow down your speed, bringing muscle, not momentum, to the movement.
- Take a day of rest between strength training to repair the body.
- Wear proper shoes to provide a stable base of support for the body.

On-the-Wall Reminders

- Hydrate and fuel the body before climbing for a successful ascent.
- Choose a partner whom you trust to hold the end of your rope. Make sure it's someone you know and not someone you just met. Your life is in his or her hands.
- Wear proper shoes that are made for climbing.
- Wear a proper climbing harness.
- Listen to your body and take a break when you need one.
- When bouldering, use a spotter when necessary.

Chapter 12
For More Information

Web Sites
www.rockandice.com
www.climbing.com
www.indoorclimbing.com
www.planet-rock.com

Magazines
Climbing
Rock and Ice

Books
The Complete Rock Climber by Malcolm Creasey
How to Rock Climb by John Long

References

Bender, Mark. 1996. *The Supple Workout Abs and Back*. New York: Barnes and Noble Books, Duncan Baird Publishers.

Chu, Donald A. PhD. 1992. *Jumping into Plyometrics*, 2nd ed. Illinois: Human Kinetics.

Craig, Colleen. 2003. *Abs on the Ball*. Vermont: Healing Arts Press.

Creasey, Malcolm, N. Shepherd, N. Banks, N. Greshem, and R. Wood, 1999. *The Complete Rock Climber*. New York: Lorenz Books, Anness Publishing Limited.

Grant, S., V. Hynes, A. Whittaker, T. Aitchison, 1996. "Anthropometric, strength, endurance and flexibility characteristics of elite and recreational climbers." *Journal of Sports and Science*. August 14(4):301-9.

Irmischer, B.S., C. Harris, R.P. Pfeiffer, M.A. DeBeliso, K.J. Adams, K. G. Shea, 2004. "Effects of a knee ligament injury prevention exercise program on impact forces in women." *Journal of Strength and Conditioning Research*. November 18(4):703-7.

Matavuji, D., M. Kukolj, D. Ugarkovic, J. Tihanyi, S. Jaric, 2001. "Effects of plyometric training on jumping performance in junior basketball players." *Sports Medicine and Physical Fitness*. June 41(2):159-64.

McBride, J.M., T. Triplett-McBride, A. Davie, R.U. Newton, 2002. "The effect of heavy- vs. light-load jump squats on the development of strength, power, and speed." *Journal of Strength and Conditioning Research*. February 16(1):75-82.

Mermier, C.M., R.A. Robergs, S.M. McMinn, V.H. Heyward. 1997. "Energy expenditure and physiological responses during indoor rock climbing." *British Journal of Sports Medicine*. September 31(3):224-8.

Quaine, F., L. Vigouroux, L. Martin, 2003. "Finger flexors fatigue in trained rock climbers and untrained sedentary subjects." *International Journal of Sports Medicine*. August; 24(6):424-7.

Sheel, A.F., 2004. "Physiology of sport rock climbing." *British Journal of Sports Medicine*. June, 38 (3):355-9.

Testa M., B. Debu, 1997. "Three dimensional analysis of variations of the forces associated with the climbing task in adolescents." *Archives of Physiology and Biochemistry*. September, 105(5):496-506.

Thompson, Clem W., 1989. *Manual of Structural Kinesiology, 11th ed.* Missouri: Times Mirror/Mosby College Publishing.

Watts, P.B., 2004. "Physiology of difficult rock climbing." *European Journal of Applied Physiology*. April 91(4):361-72.

William, Sheel A., N. Seddon, A. Knight, D.C. McKenzie, D. E. Warburton, 2003. "Physiological responses to indoor rock-climbing and their relationship to maximal cycle ergometry." *Medicine and Science in Sports and Exercise*. July 35(7):1225-31.